The
Shift

ALSO BY TORY JOHNSON

Fired to Hired:
Bouncing Back from Job Loss to Get to Work Right Now

Spark & Hustle:
Launch and Grow Your Small Business Now

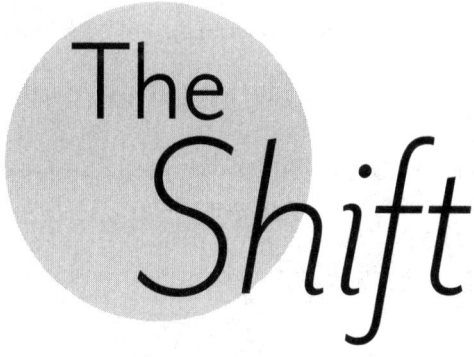

The Shift

How I Finally Lost Weight and Discovered a Happier Life

TORY JOHNSON

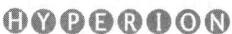

HYPERION

New York

To Barbara Fedida
for telling me what I needed to hear

All photos courtesy of Emma, Jake, and Nick Johnson.

Copyright © 2013 Tory Johnson

All rights reserved. No part of this book may be used or reproduced in any manner whatsoever without the written permission of the Publisher. Printed in the United States of America. For information address Hyperion, 1500 Broadway, New York, New York 10036.

Johnson, Tory.
The shift: how I finally lost weight and discovered a happier life/
Tory Johnson.—First edition.
pages cm.
ISBN 978-1-4013-2492-6
1. Johnson, Tory—Health.   2. Overweight women. 3. Weight loss.
4. Women—Health and hygiene.   5. Self-care, Health. I. Title.
RC552.O25J64 2013
613.2'5—dc23
2013011429

FIRST EDITION

10 9 8 7 6 5 4 3 2 1

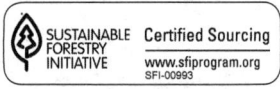

SUSTAINABLE FORESTRY INITIATIVE   Certified Sourcing
www.sfiprogram.org
SFI-00993

THIS LABEL APPLIES TO TEXT STOCK

We try to produce the most beautiful books possible, and we are also extremely concerned about the impact of our manufacturing process on the forests of the world and the environment as a whole. Accordingly, we've made sure that all of the paper we use has been certified as coming from forests that are managed, to ensure the protection of the people and wildlife dependent upon them.

Contents

Acknowledgments

I am grateful to Heidi Krupp, who believed in my idea for this book and turned it into so much more.

Many thanks to Ellen Archer, who said yes over a fun breakfast, and her talented team at Hyperion led by Elisabeth Dyssegaard, Kristin Kiser, and Ruth Pomerance; marketing and PR dynamos Christine Ragasa, Betsy Hulsebosch, and Bryan Christian; art directors Georgia Morrissey and Shubhani Sarkar; and editorial assistant Lauren Shute.

To my champions at ABC News—Diane Sawyer, Robin Roberts, Barbara Fedida, Margo Baumgart, Liz Cho, and Laura Zaccaro. No girl has better friends.

I'm grateful to Alex Hall and Gianna Fata for making the

trains run on time in our office—and staying cool amid the chaos.

And to my family: thank you for your patience, which I know I test at times, and for your enduring love, which I cherish always.

Prologue

This is not a diet book. I'm not a doctor, nutritionist, or trainer. I'm just a woman with a happy family and a successful career who lost a lot of weight in one year and, in the process, gained a level of confidence and self-respect unlike anything I'd known before.

You don't have to join a plan, make a salad, or stare down a scale—at least not today. But what you must do is start thinking that losing weight once and for all is completely and totally doable—and not impossible.

When you lose weight, especially a lot of weight like I have, everyone wants to know the secret. We—women, especially—are eager to discover the plan or program that will make the pounds melt off and stay away, hopefully forever. This book is my answer to literally thousands of women who have emailed after watching me on TV, stopped me on the street, and even chatted in restaurant bathrooms with one simple question: "Tory, how'd you do it?"

For more than a dozen years, I have taught women how to launch and advance their careers and make their professional and financial goals a reality. All the while, I was hanging on to the one dream that for me had never come true: I wanted to lose weight. I longed to see a number on the scale that said I was as healthy and happy on the outside as I felt on the inside. Most of all, I was desperate to move on. I hoped to wake up one New Year's morning with a list of resolutions that did not begin and end with dieting.

There's so much we don't control in life: being hired or fired, slumping economies, and unexpected setbacks. I spent decades under the misperception that my weight was just another thing beyond my control. I hated it. I tried and failed at diets, and I also believed that the diets failed me. My weight, and my life, didn't change until the moment I realized that *what I put in my head is far more important than what I put in my mouth.* That is what *The Shift* is all about.

After years of dieting, guilt, shame, and frustration, it took one frank conversation for me to make the Shift. I hope this book will be that spark for you.

MONTH 1

The Conversation

This day is going to suck.

It's Tuesday, December 20, 2011, a cold, dark winter morning. Having given up on a good night's sleep, I make my way into the shower. Today, I am meeting with Barbara Fedida, senior vice president for talent and business at ABC News. She is the highest-ranking woman in the news division, and I'm a contributor on *Good Morning America*. It's my first time having a one-on-one with Barbara, and I am fairly confident that there is only one item on the agenda: my weight. I think she plans to tell me that I am too fat to be on TV and that I must slim down. I am panicked because I don't just like my job, I love it and want to keep it for a long time.

With a towel perched on my wet head, I take in the quiet of the early morning. This is my safe haven: a three-bedroom apartment on the Upper West Side, a storied New York neighborhood that has been featured in movies ranging from *Annie Hall* to *Spider-Man*. Each room is filled with the people (and the dog) I love. My husband, Peter, is asleep in our bed. Friends say that he's a cross between George Clooney and Russell Crowe. I can see that, but he also has a wit and warmth that is all his own. He is my champion and best friend. If he were awake, he'd be giving me the pep talk of the century. He's always telling me how beautiful I am, and I am so grateful. But I know that no matter what he sees or says, this meeting is about my weight and I've got to steel myself for what lies ahead.

My family has supported me in my ongoing battle of the bulge, but I am the only fighter on this field. Gaining a few pounds in his forties hasn't hurt Peter's looks at all. Men are lucky that way. Down the hall, my fourteen-year-old twins, Jake and Emma, are sleeping. No weight problems there, and yet I worry that if I can't get my act together and overhaul my diet and my body, I will pass along my legacy of being overweight and the mental burden that comes with constantly struggling with your size.

I stare in my closet, frantically pulling pieces off the rack, wondering what outfit will give me the best illusion of thinness for this meeting. My closet has two bars. The eye-level shelf is for the things that fit no matter what size I am: shoes and bags in all the designer labels that I have worked so hard to afford. The other rack holds the black clothes that fit—Gap, Banana Republic, Talbots, Eileen Fisher. They don't make high-end designer stuff in my size.

I want a superhero costume, something bulletproof to protect me from the blow that I know is coming. Instead, what I grab is uninspiring at best: black wool pants and a black silk shirt, and I put them on with all the courage and hope that I can muster, which is not much right now. I'm so tired of this, of never really being happy with the way I look, no matter where I shop or how much I spend on clothing. I'm sick of the mind games I play, trying to convince myself that I'm not really *that* fat, that plenty of people weigh a lot more than I do, that America is in the midst of an obesity epidemic, that I am in good company.

My office is just fourteen blocks from my home, and when I get there I find the first of several emails from Barbara's assistant. With each one, the venue for our meeting becomes more depressing. First, it's Le Pain Quotidien, the French bistro nearby that specializes in coffee and buttery croissants for breakfast. Then it's Barbara's office at ABC News near Lincoln Center: she is so busy but really wants to meet today. Finally, it's the ABC cafeteria. Oh, great. I'm to be humiliated over a Styrofoam cup of coffee as *GMA* colleagues stroll by and guess *exactly* why Barbara has summoned me.

I have survived not one but three anchor teams at *GMA*: Charlie Gibson and Diane Sawyer, Diane and Robin Roberts, and now Robin and George Stephanopoulos. Not one of them has ever said a word to me about my weight. In fact, the bosses routinely praise my work, which enables me to think that a job well done means they're willing to overlook the obvious. But I'm not naive: I have been around television news long enough to know that thinness rules. My fit colleagues underscore that truth.

I arrive a few minutes early to scope out the scene. Barbara walks in on time wearing a fitted brown sweater that complements her bouncy brown hair. If she's wearing any makeup, it's very little. There is an effortless beauty to her, a trait she shares with many women in TV news.

We pass through the breakfast display—breads and muffins, cold cereal, eggs, bacon.

"What would you like?" Barbara asks.

Clearly, she's testing me to see if I'll bite—literally.

I opt for only a bottle of water. She grabs coffee. We find a table.

I deliberate: Take off my coat or leave it on? It adds bulk but also hides bulges. I remove it but keep it on my lap, thinking I'll fool her.

I keep watching the clock. We spend fifty minutes catching up, talking about everything but the matter at hand: our kids, New York City schools, husbands, and *GMA*'s ratings surge. We talk about how some women lack assertiveness in their careers. Barbara is funny and smart, like a character in a Nora Ephron movie. I marvel at her confidence. It could be just another great conversation with one of the many savvy women I've met over the years in network news, except I am aware of the fact that Barbara is not here to bond with me. She is warm, but she is also extremely direct. I know I am about to get it. Then I do.

"You don't look as good as you could," she says, smoothly changing the topic. "I don't think your clothing does you any favors."

In an instant, the blood rushes to my head. I feel slightly faint. My palms become sweaty and I start to twist my wedding ring, a nervous tic I've never once experienced before now. My mouth is dry. I try to remain composed even though I'm freaking out.

I'm wondering if anyone is watching us. It doesn't matter that no one I know is around. I'm certain that Barbara is starting out slowly and will soon move in for the kill: *How could you expect to be on TV when you've let yourself go? Don't you have any self-respect? You knew this day would come, right?*

But she says none of that. Instead, Barbara offers to connect me with Sandy, a stylist who helps women make smart wardrobe choices.

I'm staring blankly at her on purpose. I'm not going to make her job easy by giving her even a hint that I know my weight is a problem, that although I can easily and happily talk to millions of viewers on TV, dressing for my segment is an ongoing challenge. Finally, I crack a smile and say as cheerfully as I can, "Sure, that sounds great. I'd be happy to meet Sandy. I'd love her help."

This is a lie. Unless Sandy has a magic wand that will whisk away the pounds, I doubt she can do any good.

But Barbara is not done. "I always feel better when I work out. Exercise gives me so much energy," she presses, mildly, neither asking if I exercise nor ordering me to.

I could tell her the whole sordid story about how much I hate breaking a sweat and how I haven't taken a gym class since elementary school, about how in junior high a kid named Brian called me a fat cow when I corrected his answer and how the whole class, even the teacher, erupted in laughter. But that would go against rule number one: I do not discuss my weight with anyone except Peter. I would never share the anxiety I have about my size with people I work with, let alone someone who has the power to fire me.

Barbara continues talking as if she and I are old friends and as if everything she brings up, from her favorite spin class to the flattering effect of V-neck sweaters, is just girlish chitchat. I stare at her BlackBerry, praying for it to ping and summon her back to her office upstairs. *Please, God, give her a crisis. Please, God, let this be over.* But there is no such relief. At exactly the one-hour mark, Barbara wraps up our meeting. Numbly, I thank her for caring enough to have this chat and tell her that I look forward to meeting Sandy, which I do not. At all. We hug good-bye and wish each other a happy holiday. It is five days before Christmas. After six happy years on TV, I feel like somebody just put a lump of coal in my stocking.

As I walk quickly down the escalator and out the door onto West Sixty-Sixth Street, I try to assess the damage. I did not cry. Advantage Tory. She didn't put me on the spot, humiliate me, or embarrass me. Three points for Barbara. I marvel at how slick she was. She did not threaten me. Not once did she call me fat, say I had to lose weight, or even hint that my job was in jeopardy. The words "fat," "overweight," or "obese" never came up. But I also take her words for the clear warning shot they are meant to be: lose weight or else.

What the F am I going to do?

A New Kind of Wow

2

As the cab zips up Central Park West, I hear Barbara's words over and over again in my head. The reality is still sinking in on how precariously close I am to losing all of this, the well-paying TV gig at a place where I have worked so hard to be successful. If my waistline doesn't physically shrink—and fast—that's exactly what will happen. And what's worse, everyone who knows me will know why. Because I am fat. Period. And if I get dumped by ABC News, I will not only be full of shame, but my weight will surely make it all but impossible to get another job in television. It's a small, insular world. They all talk and compare notes. "Yeah, she's good but . . . fat."

I roll down the window, gasping for air. It occurs to me that it feels like I have been holding my breath, during and since the entire meeting. You know how on planes they say to secure your oxygen mask before your child's or anyone else who might need assistance? Talking to Barbara about my physical appearance was like being on a plane with no available oxygen. Every time I flash back to our meeting, it was like Barbara was this beautiful, calm flight attendant and I was on a plane that was losing pressure. I can see her—pretty, capable, reassuring—telling me to please secure my mask. But I am so panicked that I can barely move in my chair. All I can think is, *There's no air. I cannot breathe. There's no air.*

For years, an inner voice convinced me that I didn't take care of myself because I was too busy taking care of everyone else. But now a switch has been flipped. It wasn't just that I had to lose weight for cosmetic reasons. It was deeper, truer, and more powerful than that. I had to take care of myself because there was no way I could continue to take care of my family until I got rid of what was literally and metaphorically weighing me down.

Too many of us care for others while we neglect ourselves. It's as if we're on a plane with no air and we forget to put the oxygen mask on ourselves first. Good food is oxygen. Exercise is oxygen. Self-care is oxygen. But we deny ourselves these essentials because we don't believe we have the time. Plus, the needs of everyone else are so demanding. So the pounds pile on or the scale stays stuck on a number that is bothersome.

For most of us, when we hit a certain weight, it doesn't mean we are sloths or we lack willpower, it means that we are running on empty. In the first few hours after my conversation with Barbara, I didn't have a fully articulated vision of how I would change my body or how changing my body would change my life. But I felt that she had pointed out to me that I was running around without an oxygen mask, even though oxygen was readily available. *Even before I lose a single pound, the very first Shift I make is to pause and just breathe.*

As the taxi bobbed and weaved through traffic, I couldn't believe that my public career was about to end because of what I had always imagined was my private battle with the scale. It had always been my dream to work in network news, and I was so focused and so determined that I landed a summer internship at ABC News the summer after my freshman year of college, despite the fact that most spots went to juniors and seniors.

The next summer, when a full-time assistant left ABC's newsmagazine *20/20*, I dropped out of Emerson College and took her place. For more than a year I helped promote Barbara Walters and her newsmaker specials, and I got to know the correspondents: Stone Phillips, Lynn Sherr, and John Stossel. NBC News recruited me, and I jumped to the rival network. I worked hard and fell in love with everything about the news industry: the pace, the urgency, the immediacy, just being in the know and among the first to hear what's happening in the world.

When I left network news a few years later—truth be told, I was fired when the new boss at NBC cleaned house—I knew I had to get back in the news game someday, somehow. By then it was in my blood. But it took me years to do it. After detours into cable and publishing, I made my first major shift from employee to entrepreneur by launching my own business hosting career fairs for women. That led me to pitch my first idea to *Good Morning America*—a job search segment on how to make extra money during the holidays. It was a hit, and I was asked to come back again and again until I became the official workplace contributor. Almost two years ago, I segued into my current gig at *GMA*, a fun "Deals & Steals" segment where every week I secure exclusive deals on cool products for the show's viewers to save big bucks. I love it, my bosses love it, and viewers love it too. Most important, it's my spot in a field I'm so passionate about: network news. I thought it had been going so well that my talent trumped my weight. But suddenly everything was in jeopardy.

Despite the fact that I am a go-to problem solver for friends, family, and colleagues, now that my own career was on the line, I didn't know where to turn for advice or how I was going to fix this. I had always struggled with my weight. I thought that a lifetime of plus-sized pants was simply my destiny. Now someone had suggested that things, my body, could be different. It felt like a threat, but somewhere underneath all the panic and the shame, it also felt like an opportunity.

I had to lose a lot of weight. And let's just say, for argument's sake, that I could do it. How much was enough? My breath caught again as I thought about the daunting task ahead. I didn't need to drop ten or twenty or even thirty pounds. Just to fall into "normal" range on those maddening body mass index charts, I needed to shed at least fifty. But to look good on TV, it was probably even more than that. I hadn't lost more than eighteen pounds in the last thirty years. How would I lose eighty? The thought sent me into another tailspin. My heart was beating fast and I felt slightly faint. Maybe a little nauseated too. The cab really couldn't get home fast enough. By the time the driver turned left onto West Eighty-Sixth Street, I was desperate to get into my third-floor apartment, close the bathroom door, and cry. And that's just what I did.

It takes a lot to make me weep. I have to feel like I'm at my wits' end, totally helpless and lost. I don't allow myself to feel that way very often, but when I do, the floodgates open. This was one of those rare moments. After the meeting I didn't even have the strength or composure to go back to my office. I spent the day sobbing in peace.

Later, after I'd shed enough tears, Peter tried to comfort me. He's good at that, zeroing in on what's bothering me, then working on a plan to address it. I do the same for him.

I met Peter when I was the publicist for *Dateline* and he was *USA Today*'s TV columnist. One of my primary duties was to convince media writers to promote *Dateline* stories and profile the show's anchors and correspondents, so I made it my mission to win him over and get ink in his newspaper. We got to know each other over the phone and spent many hours talking—him in Arlington, Virginia, me in New York. Our conversations quickly moved from work to personal stuff. He was sixteen years older than me—a real man!—and his marriage was ending. I was instantly taken by his sharp sense of humor. Nobody could make me laugh more than Peter. We'd met only a handful of times in person in New York and once at a TV conference in Pasadena, California. So I was flabbergasted when one day Peter announced he was in love with me. I wondered if it was some cruel joke: What could this "normal" man possibly see in me, a fat girl? It never occurred to me that I was more than my body type. It's one of the things that Peter taught me early on.

We were married a year later on a beautiful evening in early summer at Arqua, a small, upscale Italian restaurant in Tribeca, surrounded by family and friends. Eight-year-old Nick, Peter's son, was his best man. I wore navy because I was convinced I would look like a blimp in a white wedding dress. I really wanted to wear black, my standard color, but Stella, my future mother-in-law, told me it would be too reminiscent of a funeral. Eager to please her from the beginning, I happily agreed to this compromise.

Now, seventeen years later, with our beagle, Marly, asleep at the end of our bed, Peter peppers me with questions about my meeting. Having covered the TV news industry until leaving *USA Today* in 2007, he knows how important it is for on-air talent to look their best. We both know that virtually everyone who appears on TV is even thinner in person. He is under no illusion that Barbara's chat with me was anything but a do-this-or-else conversation and not simply an offer to get me new clothes and a haircut. He knows that the financial implications of my losing the *GMA* gig would be substantial since I am the primary breadwinner in our house. But, as my husband, his first priority is to make sure I'm okay.

He eases in with leading questions.

"Was it her place to even discuss this issue?" he asks.

"Of course," I say. "If someone doesn't look or act right on-air, it's definitely Barbara's responsibility to confront them and kick ass if necessary. Every network has people like her. I'm just relieved she's given me a chance and not the boot."

"Why did she beat around the bush instead of spitting out what she meant?" he prods.

"I guess you can't just come out and tell someone she's fat." I shrug. "Or maybe it's just that she's a graceful woman. Why use a blow torch when a lighter makes the same point?"

We sit in silence for a few minutes as Peter stares at me, trying to pinpoint where I'm hurting and how much damage has been done.

"Is there any part of you that's insulted?" he asks.

"No," I tell him pointedly, "I appreciate what she has done."

He fires off other adjectives—"hurt," "furious," "livid"?—to see if I'm stuck on semantics. I remain firm in my respect for her.

"For once, someone has told me what I need to hear in a way that lets me know the consequences of doing nothing," I explain. "Yet she did it subtly, with class." Tears well up in my eyes again. "I'm grateful to her because my weight is the one thing that I have never come to grips with, but now I'm going to finally figure it out."

Peter has heard me talk many times about tackling my weight once and for all—and he's seen me fail every time. He thinks I'm still in shock and that I must be suppressing how I really feel.

He may be right. I've certainly cycled through so many emotions in the last twelve hours, but as I lie in bed as Peter falls asleep, I feel the stirrings of something, a sensation I haven't felt before. Yes, my talk with Barbara was mortifying and embarrassing, but also something potentially life altering and profound. Big. A moment that will propel me on a different course. For forty-one years I've rotated through fad diets and seesawed between denial and acceptance, and now I feel the seeds of an unfamiliar emotion, at least when it comes to weight loss: determination. Twelve hours ago, sitting in the ABC cafeteria, I thought I'd be crying myself to sleep. But now there are no more tears. Instead, I'm surprised to find that I actually feel a tiny tinge of excitement coupled with resolve. *I can do this,* I think. This time can be different. *It has to be.* Fat is my tobacco. It is my alcohol. I tell my kids not to smoke or drink, yet what I've done to myself is no better. I'm not fat by chance. This is a choice. And it's a choice I no longer wish to make.

The next morning I wake up confident that I am about to change my life, and my body, for good. Yet, it didn't take long for temptation to creep in: I still have my same old cravings for a toasted everything bagel with all the fixings. I remind myself that my cravings aren't my crime; it's the nonstop giving in to them that has taken such a toll. I won't do that today.

Peter is in the kitchen cooking turkey bacon and scrambled eggs for the kids. It smells good. I'd like to join them in there, nibbling at their plates while slathering my bagel with cream cheese. You could blindfold me and walk me forty paces away from our kitchen, and I could get to the bagels, take a knife out of the kitchen drawer, find the cream cheese in the fridge, and slice a tomato—all without a bump or a bruise. But I remind myself that I have made a commitment to change and that I will never get to where I long to be if I give in to my old patterns and habits. I am not on autopilot anymore. I must be a lean(-thinking), clean(-eating) Shifting machine. I kiss the kids good-bye, and I head to the office, stopping along the way to pick up a small container of Greek yogurt.

In addition to my work on *Good Morning America*, I run two businesses that empower women in the workplace: Women For Hire, which helps women get hired by large companies, and Spark & Hustle, which provides valuable tools and strategies to women entrepreneurs. I interact with tens of thousands of women each year. This means, among other things, that five days out of five, when I sit down at my desk and turn on my computer, I face a nonstop stream of email and correspondence.

I am still craving that everything bagel with cream cheese. I have been up for hours and I still haven't eaten. I'm not hungry, per se, but I am used to my morning meal. The temptation to just toss the yogurt and get a bagel is great. But instead, before I dive into work, before I start eating and multitasking, I open the container and scoop a creamy bite into my mouth. This is not what Oprah calls an aha moment. There is no revelatory "if only I'd known how delicious this healthy food was, I would've made better choices all along." I know what yogurt tastes like and I'm not a huge fan. What *is* an aha moment is that when I'm done, I am full and I am satisfied and, most important, I am not feeling guilty.

Maybe it's because it is December 21 and all around me New York City is tinseled and glittering, like a scene out of a Christmas movie. But as I throw the yogurt container away, I feel like I have received my first Shift Gift: *Food, for me now, is fuel. It does not have to be amazing, entertaining, or exciting.* Each meal does not have to be like a trip to the county fair or a fantasy segment of *Top Chef.* I have had enough "Wow!" meals to last a lifetime. I want a different set of "wows" now. I want "Wow! You've lost a lot of weight!" comments from my colleagues and friends. I want the "Wow!

I never thought I'd fit into this size pants" feeling when I enter a department store dressing room. I want the quiet "Oh my goodness, wow!" of stepping on the bathroom scale and seeing a number that does not make me flinch, a number that makes me feel as strong and healthy as I long to be.

The Road Trip

3

Anyone who has ever successfully lost weight knows that there is no such thing as a straight road. My Shift, while immediate and powerful, has its own early detour. Every year, my family takes a trip during Christmas break. The first year, we flew to Phoenix, then drove from Sedona to Las Vegas, soaking up the mountains and hues of the beautiful Southwest. The second year, we opted for the Pacific Northwest, starting in Seattle and driving through Portland, Oregon, to San Francisco. This year, we are heading south on a two-thousand-mile drive from New York City to Nashville and back.

Although our friends repeatedly warn us of the drama of

adolescence, Peter and I wake up daily, ever so thankful that even with the rush of hormones and the social pressures, Emma and Jake remain as warm, down-to-earth, inquisitive, and friendly as ever. Seeing this great country through their eyes has become the holiday gift that I enjoy the most.

And yet . . . two thousand miles in a car can be a long slog through the land of fatty food, sugar, and carbs. How many times had we found ourselves on the road, each rest-stop break accompanied by a swing through the on-site McDonald's, Burger King, Taco Bell, and Quiznos?

Our Honda Pilot inevitably becomes a mobile snack shack, filled with burgers, cheesesteaks, White Cheddar Smartfood Popcorn, salty pretzels, Häagen-Dazs ice-cream bars, and gooey, warm Otis Spunkmeyer chocolate chip cookies. We each have our special favorites. I crave York Peppermint Patties. Peter is hooked on Sweetarts. Jake is obsessed with Caramellos or anything that combines milk chocolate and caramel. Emma's not into candy but is content with a bag of chips.

The night before we leave, I announce to Peter and the kids, with an enthusiasm that I don't fully feel, that this road trip will be different: I will make better choices and eat less. My family, to put it mildly, is unimpressed.

Jake says, "Mom . . . Why don't you just start jogging with Uncle David in the spring?"

That's my son. Sweet. In his eyes, I'm just Mom. He doesn't understand that I weigh *a lot*. And the chances of me starting a jogging program with my greyhound-like athletic younger brother are about the same chances of me being drafted for a season of *Dancing with the Stars.*

Emma is a little savvier. "Mom," she says. "I love that you want to take care of yourself. But you know that we're not going to Seattle where you can live on fresh fish and salads and there's a vegan café on every other corner. We are going to Nashville. I think they make you sign a fried chicken pledge as soon as you cross the state line."

Peter rolls his eyes. "Come on, it's the holidays. New Year's is just eleven days away. You can start your diet then."

I knew in my gut that for me, there was no turning back. I couldn't put off the Shift because it wasn't a diet that would start on a particular day and maybe incorporate some cheat days until eventually it winnowed out. This was my new life. In order to Shift, I needed to build momentum, no matter how slight. Even if it meant I ate half a Happy Meal at every rest stop, I needed to make sure that every single day represented a step toward the woman I was determined to be.

I was sympathetic to Peter's skepticism. He'd been through this before and knew that I could be tough to live with when I was dieting, especially when he was not doing it with me. And on this trip, he had no plans to cut back on *anything.* But this wasn't about him. Or the kids. In the past, when I'd gone on a diet, I'd depended heavily on their approval and support. I needed them to help me "be good." But here it was, another Shift Gift: *Losing weight isn't about being good; it's about being good to myself.* It was so simple and yet so powerful. It wasn't a diet that I was desperate to start. What I wanted and needed to start right away was the process of being good to myself.

Still, knowing what the next two weeks would look like, I made a pact with myself. Actually, it was a compromise: from that day through the end of our trip on December 31, I would eat significantly less. I'd skip appetizers and talk someone into sharing entrées. If I were starving, I'd sneak a bite of what they were eating. No massive cheating. But I wouldn't impose my new regimen on the rest of the family because they didn't have to sacrifice on this trip. This was my battle, not theirs.

We get going early in the morning on December 24. As we make our way south along crowded stretches of I-95, I day-dream about all the junk food in our kitchen cabinets, the plus-sized clothes in my closet, my poor food choices dating back to elementary school, and my lifelong dislike of the number on the scale. Although I haven't yet lost an ounce, I know that my conversation with Barbara has roused from within me a level of determination I did not know existed. It's almost as if I am experiencing my future weight loss as a real *loss* and I am cycling through the stages of grief. I am past denial about my weight and I am firmly ensconced in anger. In my head, I blame some people for making me fat, others for calling me so.

My mood darkens at these thoughts, then suddenly brightens when the kids and Peter start belting out Top 100 songs and singing along to the corny Christmas tunes playing on

-the radio. We all wish that Peter's eldest son, Nick, had joined us on this trip.

Nick came to live with us when he was eleven, just shortly after the twins were born. They've only ever known our home to include him. Despite the age difference, all three of our kids are very close. When Nick left for college, he still spent school breaks and summer vacations at home. And after graduation, he lived with us for two more years. I've heard parents complain about boomerang kids, but for us the years Nick spent at home after college were heaven. Jake and Nick watched sports, went to pro games, and played in the park. Emma, who was in junior high when Nick returned, was so cute with him. She considered it her duty to give Nick advice about fashion, girls, and dating.

Nick is twenty-six now. He lives in Brooklyn, where he runs his own graphic design business. At least once a week he visits Jake and Emma, and they savor every second of big brother time. Now he's off skiing with buddies for the holidays. "Come on, T, I'm too old for family road trips," Nick explained gently on the phone. He may be right, but every time Jay-Z or Adele—two of Nick's favorite artists—come on the radio, we feel his absence.

We turn down the blasting music as we pull into the first rest stop along I-95. I wait in the car while they go inside: what I don't see I can't buy. I don't trust my willpower if I get a whiff of KFC or a glimpse of TCBY with assorted candy toppings. Better to have a bite—or three—of whatever snack they get, instead of devouring my own.

．　．　．

Back on the highway, Peter and the kids dig into candy, pop-corn, and potato chips that I will not allow myself to have. Staring out the window, I notice as we pass other cars that not every family is stuffing their faces. I see women my age read-ing, watching videos, or sleeping. I know America is getting fatter, but not everyone is. I read somewhere recently that Americans have cut back on their sugar intake by 7 percent in the last four years. It's not of *The Biggest Loser* proportions, but it is significant. I want to make the leap from people who are part of the problem to those who are finding solutions.

Later, during quiet times when Peter is focused on the road and the kids are dozing or listening to their iPods, I make mental notes, mapping out a blueprint of how I'm going to succeed this time—when I've always failed before.

One moment, I'm thrilled that I am finally acting to cor-rect years of unhealthy behavior.

The next moment, I'm disgusted that I've allowed my weight to get so far out of control.

Then I'm terrified I'll flunk again. How will this be differ-ent? How will I avoid the things that tripped me up before? What will keep me motivated?

When I am not looking out the window obsessing about these questions, I flip through a stack of magazines—*O, The Oprah Magazine, More, InStyle, Vogue, Marie Claire*—and I imagine myself like the fortysomethings who fill their pages. Halle Berry, Rachel Weisz, Mariska Hargitay, Naomi Watts. A generation ago, being in your forties meant pulling back from caring about your looks. But these women remind me that fortysomething can be hot. I'm not crazy enough to think that I'll look like any of these stars. But I know that there is a level of beautiful that is entirely achievable for me and now is the time for me to do what it takes to get there. I envision myself on Dr. Oz's couch talking about my dramatic weight loss as women in the audience hang on my every word.

We arrive in Nashville about twelve hours after passing through the Lincoln Tunnel, which Peter proclaims a land speed record. We got a great deal on a large suite at the Hermitage, the iconic hundred-year-old downtown hotel. If I'm not going to pig out, at least I'll sleep in a really nice bed.

We're all tired after the trip and decide to have dinner downstairs in the Capitol Grille. "Good evening, Mr. Johnson," the waiter says in fine southern tradition, welcoming only Peter as he hands him a wine list. He has ignored me, which irks me more than it should, but I'm hungry and anxious about what to eat. Emma and Jake crack up: they know Peter does his part, but I bring home the bacon. My heart races a bit as I look over the menu. Luckily the restaurant offers a range of healthy options. Me and healthy eating: what an oxymoron. Peter orders delicious-looking short ribs, which come with inky-black gravy, garlic mashed potatoes, and greens flecked with pancetta. I could devour his plate. Jake has pork, Emma pecan-crusted chicken. I choose grilled fish—and ask for the sauce on the side.

"Potatoes or rice?" the waiter asks.

"Both," I'm dying to blurt out. Instead, I ask for extra vegetables. I don't order dessert, but I do sample Peter's and Jake's.

Back in our room, we decide to hit the sack early, and after we turn out the lights Peter asks, "How hard was it today?"

"Hard. Super hard. It was impossible for me to think about anything but food. I ate so little, and even though I know it's not true, I feel like I'm starving right now."

He squeezes my hand.

I shake my head. More reassurances won't make the bright flashing lights in my brain that say EAT SOMETHING. EAT SOMETHING. YOU HAVEN'T EATEN ALL DAY go away.

"I don't know how I'm going to do this," I whisper.

"Go easy on yourself," he says, assuring me that I can and I will. Because I trust him, because I am beginning, somewhere deep down inside, to trust myself, I turn off the twenty-four-hour neon diner sign in my head and within a few minutes we're both asleep.

Next day. Same dilemma. Lunch. I'm scanning the menu like I'm reading the fine print of a legal document, searching for an acceptable healthy option. But this particular restaurant, the Loveless Cafe, a southern-fried institution in Music City, is not famous for lite choices. Oh, great. The menu boasts maple yams, smothered chicken, meatloaf with gravy, fried okra. I suspect that even the tap water is sugared. Jake orders iced tea and the waitress doesn't even bother asking if he wants it with or without sugar. It comes sweet. Very sweet, he says. Welcome to Nashville.

I watch waitresses bustling around with mammoth portions of deep-fried, mouth-watering goodness, all of which would ordinarily go straight to my ample thighs, belly, and ass. Who doesn't like this stuff? Just twenty-four hours into our trip and I am tempted to abandon this quest to eat healthy. Just this once, I tell myself. I'll be good every meal hereafter. I begin to justify it in my head: *I didn't have breakfast and saved calories there. I'll be really good at dinner.* I'm desperately grasping for excuses to gorge myself. But instead I reluctantly select the chef salad with oil and vinegar—akin to ordering sliced apples at McDonald's. Hardly a place to get a salad, which is why there are only a few on the menu.

"You'll regret that," Peter says, shaking his head in disgust, which is all I need to see. I flag the waitress to say I've changed my mind and order the quarter fried chicken, white meat only. "Which sides?" she asks pleasantly.

I am doomed. Or maybe it's just that I've hit the next mind-boggling stage of this journey. And so I make what amounts to a devil's bargain as I go for fried green tomatoes and white corn grits.

When the food arrives, I pick at my meal because I feel guilty. Then I decide I'll be damned: the food smells too good. I eat everything on my plate. In a heartbeat, I regret it. Ugh. I've pledged to not pig out at all this week—and I've done just that.

After lunch, driving past mansions owned by country music stars, Peter notices my brooding silence and asks what's wrong.

"I don't have the self-control to walk into places like that. It's killing me."

He's sympathetic, but reminds me that road trips are never easy eating, especially in the South where home cookin' rules. "Restaurants want to make you feel good, not lose weight," he says. "Just a few more days and we can cook at home and avoid all these menu dilemmas."

Seeing a convenience store up ahead, I ask him to stop and get me another soda, my fourth of the day. I can't bring myself to skip DP—as I've nicknamed Diet Pepsi. I have been drinking the stuff for more than twenty years. It was Diet Coke before that—until I discovered that DP tastes even sweeter. I drink five cans a day, but I prefer the fountain variety. Now I'm drinking even more from those sixteen-ounce cups to replace the sweets I'm avoiding. But in the back of my mind I know I'm going to have to cut out DP entirely. I've read time and again that aspartame, the sweetener in diet sodas, triggers appetites because your body is being tricked into thinking it's ingesting sugar, so you crave more and more. Why is this so goddamn complicated? Why is diet soda—which is marketed as the decent alternative to sugar—now the enemy?

We pass the Pancake Pantry in Hillsboro Village and Emma googles it from the backseat and learns it's the place for breakfast. The next morning, after waiting in line for

twenty minutes to be seated—a first for me for breakfast—
our table crests with eggs, pancakes, waffles, home fries, grits,
sausage, bacon, and toast. I manage to eat a single scrambled
egg, a slice of bacon, and a few bites of Jake's chocolate chip
pancakes, which he has smothered with maple syrup and
four or five pats of butter.

It's a shift of the most microscopic proportions, but I make
it. I learn to say "I'm full" when my family notices that I'm
not wiping the plate clean.

"Everything okay, Mom?" Jake asks when I leave three of
four pieces of toast on my plate.

The last thing I want to be is a buzzkill, the mom on a diet
who makes her kids feel needlessly guilty about what they're
eating. I must find a balance between being a good role
model—making sensible food choices—and denying them
food they love. What purpose would I serve by making a sour
face when Jake ordered those delicious pancakes—a dish that
he's perfectly entitled to enjoy?

We return home on New Year's Eve and I prepare to face
our bathroom scale with trepidation. It doesn't really matter
if I've gained or lost because the clock starts fresh for good
tomorrow.

We always ring in the New Year with a fun but over-the-
top feast—anything anyone wants—and Peter assures Emma
and Jake that it's the same deal this year. I feel like I'm on
death row: What to have for my Last Supper? One part of
me wants to choose a gigantic baked potato, loaded with

butter. But sweets have always been my downfall. I'd love to eat an entire chocolate cake, maybe with a side of tiramisu. Everyone encourages me to indulge.

"Go ahead, Mom. It's a special occasion!" Jake says enthusiastically, wanting me to be happy after seeing me so consciously trying to be good on vacation.

Instead, I opt for a chicken cutlet and a small salad with ginger dressing. This unfair deprivation—at least that's how I see it, even though I had just made a smart food choice— sends me into a funk. So shortly after dinner, I go to our bedroom and leave Peter and the kids to the festivities. Jake is digging into chicken wings and Emma is sampling chocolate-covered strawberries.

I am feeling more contemplative than celebratory tonight. Safely tucked in my pajamas, with Ryan Seacrest's voice echoing from the living room, I start thinking of the significance of this night: every single year for as long as I can remember, I have made my New Year's resolution to conquer my weight . . . then broken it a few days or weeks later. This time has to be different. I'm anxious but resolute. I may have failed every time before, but that doesn't mean this year can't be different. Won't be different. I've got to do it. It feels impossible, but I must summon the resolve. I think about how there are moments that happen in your life when big things change. There is before and after. Some are obvious: graduation day, your wedding night, or the birth of a first child. But some are more subtle—and this is one of them. I realize that since my talk with Barbara, something fundamental has changed for me and in my outlook on life. Forever. There is now Before Barbara and After Barbara. The specter of getting the boot from *Good Morning America* hurts more than finally dealing with this lingering weight nightmare. Dropping at least fifty pounds will be a steep challenge—the hardest thing I've ever done—but sacrificing my career over it would be harder. I will not allow that to happen.

Inspired, I jump up from bed and grab a note card from the desk and head to the bathroom. With a big sigh I step onto the scale—left foot first, then slowly, as the red line rushes to the right, I put my right foot down. I'm staring at the harsh reality, the numbers that I have let define me. In bright red ink to match the numbers on the scale, I write *12/31/11 9:48 p.m.* and the three pathetic digits onto the note card. I stare at my weight and realize that I weigh fourteen pounds more tonight than I did the morning I entered New York University Medical Center to give birth to Emma and Jake at thirty-six weeks. I shove the card into an envelope, seal it, and tuck it away. Ironically, the card I've chosen has a cupcake motif across the top. Sick. Well, by the time I pull out this card next year, cupcakes will be a distant memory, along with grilled cheese sandwiches, waffle fries, and tortellini. In their wake will be the new me.

There's a proverb that says, "Fall seven times and stand up eight." As a society, we've fallen for dozens, if not hundreds, of diets. And more often than not, we fail at them. This is not about falling in love with a diet or how many times you've failed. *The Shift happens when you say, "This time I'm not going to fall for the gimmick or the quick scheme. This time I'll stand up for my body and my health, and I will keep standing for myself, meal after meal, until I figure out my eating issues and get to my happy weight, whatever that may be."* It comes to me as clearly, quickly, and powerfully as lightning striking. And I know, in that instant, that Barbara gave me more than a warning; she gave me a gift.

I fall asleep before the ball drops in Times Square. Happy New Year to me. I am eager to wake up in 2012, the year that everything changes.

make the *Shift*

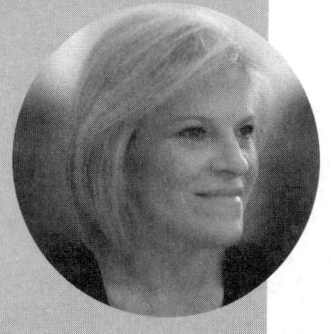

What I put in my head is far more important than what I put in my mouth.

For now, food is fuel. It does not have to be amazing, entertaining, or exciting.

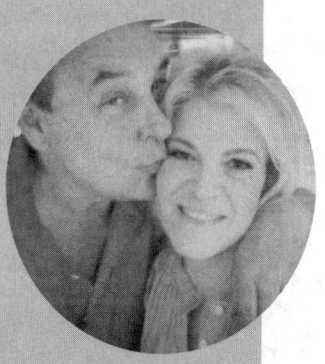

Losing weight isn't about being good; it's about being good to myself.

MONTH 2

The Cleanout

decided to clean out the kitchen cabinets. I had been good, but the temptation was too great. All the foods on my "no" list had to go. Because I knew that there would be protests from Peter and the kids, I woke up early and, trailed only by our beagle, the massive clean-out began. Dressed in comfy sweats and a tee, I started pulling stuff I would no longer eat off the shelves with the hope of donating it to a nearby food pantry. There was a bomb shelter's worth of grains: brown rice, white rice, couscous, barley, two bags of Spanish yellow rice. Enough to feed a dozen families for a month, maybe two. I took out two bags of seasoned croutons: the big chunks of toasted bread that once upon a time were the only thing that made salads

palatable to me. There was a big bag of dried cranberries—
also for salads. And a huge unopened bag of baked Cheetos.
I had convinced myself that if the Cheetos were baked they
were okay, diet food even. Not anymore. I had made the
Shift and I wanted to stop playing games with myself about
what I could or couldn't eat if I was really serious about losing the weight for good.

There was more. A box of Kudos bars with M&M'S. Out.
I pulled out two boxes of cake mix—one chocolate and one
vanilla. That reminded me not to forget the fridge: I found a
tub of Duncan Hines chocolate frosting in there, just as I
suspected. I opened the freezer, and as if it were all a big
deconstructed dessert, there were the cake's missing pieces:
two pints of ice cream. I was surprised at how easy this was,
to say "No, not now" to food before it was made, how very
different it was from sitting in a restaurant summoning the
willpower to order salad not pasta, to drink just water when
everyone else was having dessert. I reminded myself that this
was my choice. I *could* have anything in my kitchen. I *chose*
not to have it—any of it.

I turned my attention to the last cabinet. There was an
opened bag of chocolate chips for baking and an unopened
bag of peanut butter chips too. I love to bake, especially
when I am in the kitchen with Emma and Katy Perry is
blaring from the speakers, pop beats as sweet and sugary
as the confections we whipped in our big mixing bowls.
But I was Shifting, and for now, there would be no such
fun.

Emma was in her room, oblivious to the big cleanout. But Jake walked in just as I was about to toss a half-eaten jar of Nutella, his favorite. He saved it from the trash bin, mere seconds before it was history. "Whoa," he said with a scowl. "What are you doing?"

I smiled at him. "Jake, I am starting fresh."

He was not pleased. "Well, don't ditch my Nutella." Grabbing the jar protectively, he walked out of the kitchen, no doubt to alert his dad.

Moments later, Peter showed up. He was more than a little peeved that I was getting rid of things that were sealed. He'd never seen me do a cupboard overhaul, and since he is the one who does the cooking, he was afraid that I would ditch something that he wanted or needed.

I was, to put it mildly, strident. "I can't have anything in the house that might interfere with my success."

If the cleanout was a unilateral decision that I made without consulting Peter or the kids, then I was willing to take responsibility for it. For once in my life, I was going to put myself first. I needed the fresh start of a clear kitchen filled only with things that supported my quest to lose what had been weighing me down for decades. You may reach a moment like this—when something feels absolutely and categorically right for your Shift and nobody else around you fully understands. If it's not physically or emotionally hurting anyone, then I say go for it. Shift now. Apologize later.

The question is often, how? Let me give you two Shift

Gifts that seemed to come to me immediately when I became committed to this change:

1. CLARITY TRUMPS WILLPOWER.

Previously, whenever I began a diet, I approached it like a gladiator going into battle. In order to make the plan work, I would prepare to win not just the battle, but the war. And what it took to win the war—in my own imagination—was an arsenal of willpower that would help me torpedo my way through temptation after temptation until I emerged on the other side of the battlefield, slim and victorious. Similarly, whenever I saw a woman who seemed to be what I wanted to be—slim—I imagined that she was either lucky (born that way!) or else she had a vault of willpower filled with gold ingots piled sky-high, all that diet determination just sitting there.

But when I began my Shift, I approached it quite differently. I knew that I was going to stand up for myself and my health at every single meal, and that meant I didn't need a warehouse full of willpower. I didn't need to think about how I was going to possibly survive the three-day juice cleanse or the seven-day carb reduction or the twenty-one-day bikini body program. All I needed was the clarity to stay true, hour by hour and meal after meal, to my commitment.

2. THE SECRET TO SUCCESS ISN'T IN CHOOSING THE RIGHT PLAN. THE SECRET TO SUCCESS IS ACTUALLY MAKING THE SHIFT.

The second Shift Gift is that while you need a plan to lose weight, the food part doesn't have to be complicated. Just eat a lot less. If you love Weight Watchers, use the Shift to rock that out. If you're feeling curious about the Paleo diet and the Shift helps you shore up your commitment to that program, then by all means, go for it.

For my Shift, I developed a simple three-rule plan that didn't involve any particular program or specific meals. I know myself and my lifestyle. I travel a lot. I eat away from home often. In the past, when I was trying to stick to a rigid program, let's say the "Soup and Cereal" diet, I'd crumble when I didn't immediately have a soup or cereal option.

I wanted a plan that drew on what I understood about losing weight and one that I could follow anywhere. I wrote it out on a little note card, tucked it inside my purse, and carried it everywhere. My plan featured three straightforward and simple main rules:

1. Eat a whole lot less.
2. Don't exceed twenty-five carbs a day.
3. Avoid anything fake.

The first is a big one because up until a few months before my Shift, I had always eaten whatever I wanted, whenever I felt like it, and as much as I desired. Aside from dozens of short-lived diet attempts, I never placed any real food limits on myself. Now I had to consume much less, which I arbitrarily determined would be *at least half* of what I used to eat. I quickly discovered a little trick: if I could easily list everything I ate for the day in under ten seconds, I probably wasn't overeating. After a few weeks, when I reviewed what I typically ate, it became clear that it was a massive reduction.

The second rule—twenty-five carbs or less—effectively meant no white anything: no rice, bread, pasta, or sugary stuff. I also included brown carbs in the off-limits category as well, because in the past I ate so-called healthy carbs like brown rice, multigrain bread, and whole wheat pasta. Before I knew it, I was back to eating all kinds of carbs again. Same with oatmeal, granola, and smoothies. They're all offenders, just as bad for me as anything pure white. Long ago, before I knew what I was doing carb-wise, I would eat that stuff thinking it was acceptable. Wrong. I know that some people aren't fans of low-carb diets, but I have found that avoiding carbs is definitely the quickest and most effective way for me to shed pounds.

I stay within my limit by refusing to eat anything until I know the carb count. This means I now read nutrition labels on all packaged foods. In the absence of a label, I look it up online or on an iPhone app. Eventually, when I reach a healthy weight, I will add more carbs to my diet. Cutting carbs was a killer in early January, because as I weaned myself from sugar, my body begged for a baked potato, a bagel, or a twelve-pack of cupcakes. It took pausing to reflect on my goal—often several times a day—to stop me from reaching for any of it. But I did it, and within a couple of weeks, the payoff began.

My next hard-and-fast rule is nothing fake. Thankfully, I had already given up sugar-free candy and chocolate, and I'll never go back. I used to devour those treats because they satisfied my sweet tooth and because I assumed anything sugar-free couldn't hurt. I was wrong. High calorie fake food isn't a treat. With one exception: Diet Pepsi. Nothing fake also meant the end of my two-decade affair with my beloved DP. I stopped drinking it cold turkey on New Year's Eve and, to my surprise, I don't miss it. I stick to water—bottled or tap—and I sip all day. I convince myself that it curbs hunger pangs, helps flush salt from my body, and makes me feel full.

At home, I keep an oversized glass pitcher of iced water with orange or lemon slices in it near me—like they have in the lobby of trendy hotels. It looks good and tastes great. When I really need something more, I make two teeny exceptions to my no-fake commitment: I chew Dentyne Fire sugar-free gum or I reach for Target's Market Pantry Sugar Free On-the-Go Lemonade. I discovered years ago that it tasted better than other sugar-free drinks and has just five calories per serving. But one day after I poured a tall glass of it, my resident chemist, Jake, read the nutrition label and walked into the living room to tell me—quite proudly—that it contains the same fake sugar additive as in diet sodas.

"How can you drink this stuff when it's just as bad as DP?"

my fourteen-year-old asked, a bit too accusingly for my taste. "Isn't that a variation on what Dad calls 'Speaking with a forked tongue'?"

"Guilty, Your Honor, but with an explanation," I told him. "I can easily stop at one glass of this, which I never could do with DP."

Jake got that logic.

I think anytime people tackle big-ticket items in life—moving, changing careers, getting married or divorced—they do better with a plan. A step-by-step guide that outlines how they're going to get from point A to point B with their sanity in check and leaves nothing significant to chance. It doesn't have to be a long, detailed document—an index card with three rules did the trick for me. And everyone's plan will look different based on your unique challenges and circumstances. But the key is to *have* some sort of plan to get you going and to look at when things go wrong or when you begin to question whether you can actually accomplish what you set out to do.

The Birthday Party

5

We are invited to a friend's birthday party. Just the idea of facing forbidden foods for a night puts me on edge. So far, I'd been making smart choices about food. Almost two months without a single sweet, chip, or diet soda! But this night I'm anxious about confronting temptation. Plus, parties always make me nervous: What to wear to not look huge? Double anxiety. I spend more than an hour trying on outfits before choosing basic black (of course), and I stew on the drive from the Upper West Side to Chelsea. I predict that every woman will be normal-sized—and look great. Once again, I'll be the Fat One. I know we have to go to this party—and I should want to hang with people we like—but I am oh-so-tempted to dredge up some excuse, lame or not, and stay home.

"Watch," I tell Peter gloomily, "they'll serve a ton of hot hors d'oeuvres and big bowls of pasta."

"Right, but I'm sure it'll be low-carb pasta," he says, trying to inject some humor. I don't laugh and Peter senses my tension.

"You know they'll have decent options," he continues with an attitude, clearly bothered by my negativity. "But whatever they serve, you can just sample a bite or two. No reason to make a big deal out of it or get into a funk."

I let his little lecture sink in, then explain that it doesn't work that way. The food fare at all parties is toxic for anyone looking to lose weight: it's meant to be yummy, not healthy, which is why all passed appetizers taste great and are no-no's for someone in my position.

"I'll be the girl with the glass of water and a carrot stick," I say, feeling way too sorry for myself for Peter's liking.

I think to mention to him that I misspoke. With my newfound knowledge about acceptable foods, I've learned that carrots are loaded with carbs—not the best veggie for my current plan. But I hold that thought to myself to avoid getting another well-meaning but irksome pep talk from him.

We arrive at the party and are assaulted by a dizzying display of delicious-smelling hors d'oeuvres at the top of my Do Not Sample list: puffed pastries stuffed with feta cheese, spreads on crackers, cheeseburger sliders, and pigs in a blanket—all loaded with fat and carbs. I decline every offer with a fake half smile: "No thanks." I could eat everything put in front of me. But I don't.

Dinner comes about forty-five minutes later and I make the motions. I taste a bit of salad and pretend to enjoy the lasagna, but what I'm really doing is breaking it apart and moving bits around my plate to give the impression of eating. To my surprise, no one notices or seems to take any interest in how much I eat—or don't eat. I park that observation in the back of my mind and begin to watch others in the room.

I notice that all the thin people are eating slowly, putting their forks down between bites to chat or catch their breath. If I were eating this meal alone now, I'd be shoveling food into my mouth, cleaning my plate in minutes. But they're not in any hurry to finish. The portions they take for themselves are small. None of them clears everything on their plate. *They eat slowly and their portions are small.* I park this thought somewhere in my head too. How have I never recognized these things before?

Dessert is harder to resist. The birthday girl sets up an ice-cream bar with three Ben & Jerry's flavors: Phish Food, Chunky Monkey, and Cherry Garcia. I'm not into fruity ice cream, so I could care less about the last one. But Chunky Monkey is rich banana ice cream with fudge chunks and walnuts, and Phish Food is even more sinful: dark chocolate ice cream with creamy swirls of marshmallow and caramel and—hello!—fish-shaped fudge bits swimming through the whole damn thing. How to resist?

"Stop killing yourself," Peter whispers to me, exasperated. "Have a little bit."

"Screw you," I hiss, furious that he thinks enabling me is the solution. I manage to refuse the ice cream, and denying myself feels like a small victory while I watch everyone else in the room indulge.

Heading home up Tenth Avenue an hour or so later, we ride in silence. I'm upset that every social occasion seems like a threat to the Shift I am trying so hard to make; Peter is annoyed because he thinks this is old territory: me on a diet is always a downer. I remember standing in our kitchen at a party we once threw. One of our guests kept asking for espresso after espresso, which I was happy to serve him because he said he had just quit drinking. He wanted to be at our party, he told me, but found that being around booze was driving him crazy. He understood that there was no middle ground; having just a sip of alcohol in any form would derail him. Coffee helped. He is still sober today, years later. As Peter turns right onto West Eighty-Sixth Street, I come to a major conclusion: There is no middle ground for me either. Nothing in between. If I'm going to conquer this thing, it's all or nothing no matter where I am. This is about me, not about my surroundings. Parties, restaurants, office, or home—the place doesn't matter because the fight is always with me. It is a daily battle and a long war with surrender not an option.

6

Mean Girls

We get home and I stay up to watch the late news while Peter falls asleep. The phone rings, and when I answer, a voice I love greets me by asking, "So how's it going?" I smile. I keep very few secrets from my younger brother.

David and I have a special bond that goes way back. From the time he could walk he often came to me, his only sibling, to snuggle. I changed his diapers, fed him, and took him on long walks around our neighborhood when Mom was working. I protected him, gave him advice, and urged him to attend college in New York to be near me. Now, as adults, we live in the same town and constantly talk, email, and see each other. CC, as we say: constant communication.

I've told him all about the Shift and my plan to drop a lot of weight, which he knows has bothered me forever. He also knows that it's the one obstacle that has bested me time and again and he frequently gives me tips on dieting. David is a documentary filmmaker who is as gifted intellectually as he is committed physically. He ran the New York City Marathon a few years ago; he golfs with Peter, Nick, and Jake; he plays pickup basketball every weekend. He's obsessed with things like Tim Ferriss's *The 4-Hour Body*, and we joke that his newborn daughter, Charlotte, will be swinging kettlebells before she takes her first step.

"Tonight was rough," I say, launching into how hard it was to resist the hors d'oeuvres, pasta, and that outrageous ice cream.

I can hear the compassion in David's voice; he knows how challenging every second of this journey is for me. He pulls out a memory from our childhood, as if to remind me of the poor training we both received in the ways of healthy eating.

"Do you remember that our freezer was like Baskin-Robbins?" David asks. "And the first thing our friends did when they came to our house was head to the oven?"

We both burst out laughing, but before we can talk more David has to go: Charlotte just woke up and is crying.

David's mention of childhood, our freezer and the oven, prompts me to think about the origins of my compulsive eating. Our freezer was stuffed with ice cream, pizza, and assorted frozen, microwavable packages. We never used the bottom oven on our stove because it was stuffed with snacks:

Funyuns, Oreos, Chips Ahoy!, nacho-cheese-flavored Dori-
tos, Ruffles potato chips, Cheetos, and Cheez-Its. Other kids
would walk in and make a beeline for all of it, just as I did
many times a day.

I remember watching TV in my bedroom when Mom
called me to come sit with her on our brown velour couch in
the living room to announce she was pregnant. At seven
years old, and as the only child, nothing could have made me
happier than the prospect of a sibling, a real baby in the house!

We headed to McDonald's at Seventy-First Street and
Collins Avenue to celebrate. This is one of my earliest and
clearest recollections of the thousands of poor food choices
that have plagued me all my life. As a second grader, I was
already a good twenty pounds overweight, a direct result of
unhealthy eating habits. Like a lot of families, we equated
food with comfort. Good day? Celebrate with snack. Bad
mood? Nothing that a microwave pepperoni pizza can't cure.
Feeling blue? Dive into that box of chewy Entenmann's chocolate chip cookies.

That night, when my mother announced that I would soon
have a little sister or brother, I ate a Kid's Meal: hamburger,
fries, and a Coke. My addiction to sugary drinks started
early and it wasn't just soda. Throughout my childhood and
into my teen years, when I wanted to make a "healthier"
drink choice, I downed glass after glass of fruit juice, oblivious to calories or carbs. I had come to believe that anything
with fruit was healthy: Tropicana orange juice, Ocean Spray
cranberry, Welch's grape juice, and all those small Capri Sun
packages. Liquid sugar.

These were hardly the dark ages. It was the late seventies and early eighties, and people were beginning to take health and fitness seriously. Health clubs were catching on. And we lived in Miami Beach, a national wellness hot spot, where people show off their bodies, wearing as little as possible. Yet, as generous and caring as my mom has always been, in our house, we didn't talk about any connection between regular Coke, calories, and obesity. Nor did we ever talk about healthy food options or link our food choices to our expanding waistlines.

Both my parents worked full time: my father as an architect and my mother managing a children's clothing store. They came home tired, and neither had much interest in cooking, let alone whipping up complicated meals. So by default, the cooking sometimes fell to me. Over the course of my childhood, I became an expert at making packaged meals like Hamburger Helper, scalloped potatoes, and Rice-A-Roni. I fried hot dogs and ground beef, creating puddles of fat in the pan. Every meal I prepared included rice, a baked potato, or pasta for all of us: they're easy and we loved them. Who doesn't?

Once a week we would head to Flora's, a popular outdoor pizzeria, where we'd order garlic knots and cheesy pies. Every couple of days, we would stop at a local bakery for a treat: fresh corn muffins and my favorite hi-top cupcakes—chocolate cream–filled, hat-shaped towers of sugary sweet goodness.

I can practically taste a hi-top in my mouth as another embarrassing memory from childhood comes rushing back:

the day my dentist asked Mom, during a routine appointment, if she was "gaining or expecting," as if inquiring about
the weather. My mother, who was always beautiful and stylish
in my eyes, was not pregnant; David was already three. She
and I never acknowledged, much less discussed, his comment.
Instead, we headed across the street to Carvel for soft-serve
ice cream.

I think about that incident at the dentist's office often—
especially when I am shopping for clothes and I try on a
blouse that makes me look not just fat but pregnant. The
cruelty of the dentist's comment is seared in my mind: "Gaining or expecting?" All these years later, I'm still bothered by
his thoughtlessness and how often people think it's perfectly
okay to just say what's on their minds, no matter how inap-
propriate or mean.

At the reception for my grandfather's funeral, early on in
our marriage, a distant aunt who had never met Peter asked
if he was fat or just had a beer belly. He smiled at this odd
question and said, "Maybe I need to do a few more sit-ups."
He brushed it off, but I could see it hurt. I was furious. What
a heartless world where people feel free to say what they
wish about the bodies we live in—thin or not. I would never
walk into someone's home and say, "God, that couch is a
weird color," or "That lamp is awful." But many of us—
friends, family, strangers—seem to feel free in the guise of a
joke, a dig, or just casual conversation to comment on our
bodies. I find it rude and tacky.

It's a small victory for me that Peter and I use the oven in our kitchen as an actual oven, not a snack bin, but there is no doubt that I am still trapped in old habits and the humiliation associated with being fat. For a moment, I wonder what's worse: being called out about my weight by a successful network TV executive as an adult or being taunted by a classmate, as I was as a child. On some level both are a punch in the gut, and yet only one of them has prompted me to change.

Since she started high school, Emma has noticed how cruel teenagers can be. But it's primarily the girls, and most of the snarky comments revolve around who looks good and who doesn't. Having the perfect body is expected, especially among the popular crowd. To them, if your physique is anything short of a perky little Barbie body, you're a loser.

One evening as I walked in the door from work, Emma greeted me by fuming, "Kids are obsessed with physical appearance! You have no idea what it's like." I smiled, thinking about the perennial paradox of each generation thinking the previous one can't possibly understand. If she only knew.

"Emma, you can't let those girls get to you," I told her, even though I know it's much easier said than done. "You're gorgeous, smart, and sweet and, as far as I'm concerned, perfect." But the truth is she isn't stick skinny, so I decided on the spot to give her some advice that I wish I had heard when I was her age. "You know, you'd probably feel better about yourself if you lost just five pounds, which won't be hard at all if you put your mind to it," I told her.

"You think I'm fat?" she asked, bracing for a fight.

"Not at all, and you know that," I said. "You're not even close to having my high school predicament—needing to lose thirty to forty pounds—but if you lost a few pounds, I bet it'd boost your spirits. I don't want history to repeat itself."

She burst into tears because she assumed I was critical of her appearance. I assured her that was not my intention. As I soothed her, I said I wanted to be able to discuss my new regimen with her. I also told her that weight should be a subject we talk openly about instead of ignore. We hugged and she agreed. Emma is so beautiful and it breaks my heart to imagine her ever doubting it for a second. But I also know that for years people closest to me did not sound the alarm about my weight, and as a result, I became complacent and comfortable with my excuses. Emma has no real weight issues, but I hope that if I ever see her denying the self-care that she deserves, I can tenderly and clearly remind her that good food is oxygen and exercise is oxygen, and that she must take care of herself first and foremost.

I lost count of how many times Emma and I have watched *Mean Girls*. Sometimes we have our movie nights in my bedroom, but just as often we are in Emma's room, cuddled together on her queen-sized bed. She has a dream teen room: bright bubblegum-pink walls, chocolate-brown accents, her favorite teddy bears from childhood safely ensconced on a top shelf, books, framed photos, nail polishes, and necklaces scattered across her dresser.

Talking with Emma reminded me just how powerful these

"mean girl" moments in our childhoods can be. We like to think we can forget them and move on, that adulthood and maturity take away the sting, but some memories still bite. I remember always being picked last for team events in phys ed because nobody wanted the slow fat girl on their side. I hid in the bathroom during gym class, hoping that no one noticed. But they always did. Successive calls were made to my parents, who would try to get me excused: *Tory's not very athletic, so could you cut her some slack?* The leniency would last for about a week before I was ordered to climb a rope or cross the tall monkey bars or some activity at which I would usually fail and the shame would make me want to cry.

By high school, I found more creative excuses to avoid gym, because there was no chance I was changing into short shorts in an open locker room, then forced to sweat for forty minutes. I forged Mom's signature on a waiver that said a back injury prevented me from participating in the required two years of physical education. Bye-bye, PE.

Even in college, where I hoped a new set of friends might cut me some slack about my weight, it still plagued me. In my first days at Emerson, I found a letter from my petite room-mate to her father, which read: *My roommate is quite large.* It shouldn't have surprised me since it was true. But it hurt to see her describe me solely in terms of my size. I held no grudge because I very quickly learned that she was warm and thoughtful, never once treating me like anything but a normal girl. And she eventually became one of my most treasured friends.

Yet these experiences conspired to make me extremely

self-conscious. Throughout adolescence I avoided fancy parties and group get-togethers like the plague. I didn't attend a single school dance because it meant wearing a dress. Not a chance. Ditto for pool parties: no way I was putting on a bathing suit. Ever. I didn't even like to be picked up by friends in their two-door cars because it might involve climbing into the backseat, which caused anxiety: Could I squeeze through the crack if someone in the front seat didn't want to get out and move their seat forward to accommodate me?

In my own car, it was an altogether different story. It gave me the freedom to eat anything anywhere, anytime. From the day I got my driver's license, I developed a habit of pigging out at drive-throughs. When I rolled up alone to the window, I would pretend I was ordering for a few people by saying out loud, "What *was* it they wanted?" As if the clerk at the window cared. Like a secret alcoholic who hides booze in a coffee cup or takes swigs from a hidden bottle, in public and around certain friends and their body-conscious moms, I hid the truth about what I was really eating. Even as a teenager, I quickly realized that self-deception and denial played such a strong part in obesity: both became an integral part of who I was.

I found that the best way to survive in my own skin was to intentionally adopt a split personality: Outwardly, I was loud and chatty—hardly a wallflower. Not a trace of shyness. Irreverent, witty, and bursting with self-confidence. I did an excellent job of faking an image of a contented teenage girl. I was mischievous and somewhat of a rebel too.

I was so sure of myself that I once called an admissions

officer at Boston University and posed as a high school guidance counselor. I proceeded to give a friend an excellent recommendation and said she would be a valuable addition to the university. I don't know if it made any difference, but she got in and graduated four years later.

At my graduation from Miami Beach Senior High School, I handed out hundreds of marbles to my fellow seniors and asked them to give theirs to the principal as he handed them a diploma. In no time, marbles were spilling out of his pockets and rolling onto the stage floor. The entire audience laughed. My classmates gave me high fives and told me how much they loved the practical joke.

But beneath my tough exterior, I was a scared and insecure girl, deeply ashamed of being fat. I thought about it constantly and fretted about my inability to deal with it. But I did it all privately and shared none of it with anyone. Ever. To do so would be too humiliating.

Fast-forward twenty or so years, and not much has changed. Yes, I'm an adult, happily married, with wonderful kids and a great job, but inside in many ways, I am still the anxious teenager wondering what people think about me and my weight. Staying away from high school pool parties has evolved into avoiding nearly all cocktail parties and black-tie dinners, even though that's where people make enduring personal and business bonds. I'll be damned if I'm going to stick out in slacks and a blouse, the fat woman who doesn't bare a thing, while the other women are in party dresses, looking sexy and sleek.

In high school, I begged my mother to take me shopping to find something, anything, trendy that would fit on my chunky teenage body. These days, I spend my hard-earned paychecks buying clothes that cover me up, frequently conning myself into thinking I look . . . normal. And just like in high school and college, I still cringe in front of mirrors, especially full-length ones.

This trip down memory lane gets me thinking about what kept me from making the Shift until now. It comes to me: *Whenever I've thought about changing my future, I've let my past weigh me down.* If you've always been overweight like I have, or been fat for many years, it's quite a hurdle to envision living any other way. The difficulty of fixing it—fathoming even where to start—just seems too high.

These memories still haunt me even though I am committed to my Shift and, at times, the weight of the past threatens to derail me. I've hidden behind the same habits and excuses for years. I blamed my parents for making me fat and allowing me to become addicted to overeating. I blamed McDonald's for serving fattening burgers and fries. I blamed my compulsive eating on the mean kids in school, sadistic gym teachers, and even the cruel president of NBC News who fired me without warning by saying, "Tory, it's a big world out there and I suggest you go explore it."

I'm sick of dodging the blame and pinning excuses for my actions on other people and situations. I can see now how I let the comfort of complacency carry me from fragile teenager to forty-one-year-old adult, and how easy it would be to stay the course for another month or year, just as I have my whole life. But I can't. I won't. Now, as I make this simple shift in my thinking, what once seemed daunting suddenly becomes much more doable and manageable.

Emma has grown up with the benefit of a mother who is a successful entrepreneur with a fun career as a morning-show contributor as the icing on the cake. What she hasn't had is a mom who models healthy behavior with great food choices and an active lifestyle. She is fourteen years old, and there's a part of me that wants to beat myself up: *I've already failed her. She's a beautiful, healthy girl, but it's no thanks to you, Tory.* Instead, I remind myself that my kids—wanting to inspire them and be a role model for them—are powerful fuel for my Shift.

I imagine Emma and Jake fifteen years from now. They are both about to turn thirty, set in their careers, settling down with their significant others. In my head, I picture them being as close as David and I are right now. Except instead of talking about how our house was the junk-food depot for all of their friends, they are having a very different conversation.

Emma says, "Remember when Mom lost all that weight?"

Jake says, "Yeah. At first, it seemed like such a drag . . . But then it was like we were all so proud of her."

I hear Emma laughing, "And now she's a runner. Which means . . ."

Jake finishes her thought, the way twins so often do: "We

all have to do that lame Turkey Trot before we get any Thanksgiving dinner."

Emma says, "You're just mad because I beat you last year."

Jake won't be bested. "If I hadn't stopped to tie my shoe-laces . . ."

I look at Emma, all that I hope and dream for her, and I know that I can't take back the years of poor eating habits. I don't want to make casual comparisons, but I wonder if this is how an alcoholic feels when she finally gets sober. How a pill addict mom feels when she finally gets clean. Does she look at her child and want to wipe her memory clean with a wave of a magic wand the way Will Smith and Tommy Lee Jones do in *Men in Black*? I know what I feel, but I also know that this guilt is a distraction—and just like that, I let myself off the hook. What matters is that I am Shifting now. And because I know that this is not a diet or a phase or anything I can fail at, I let myself feel good about this very special Shift Gift: *The past is past.*

make the *Shift*

SHIFT WISDOM

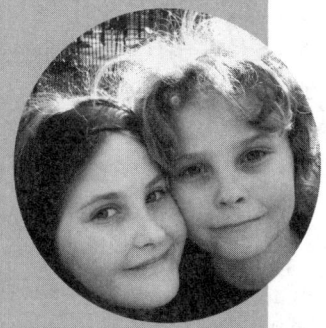

The past is past.

Clarity trumps willpower.

FUEL YOUR SHIFT

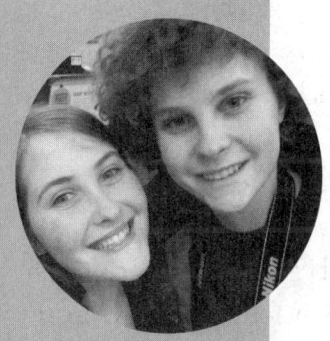

Find what inspires you. For me, the biggest inspirations are my kids: Emma, Jake, and Nick. Another is a career that I cherish.

MONTH 3

7

The First Eleven Pounds

"**E**leven friggin' pounds," I bark to Peter from the bathroom after weighing myself.

"Hey, great," he says, looking up momentarily from the *New York Post*.

"It sucks," I say, slamming the door and turning on the shower.

For sixty days and nights, I have been walking purposefully along the barren food tundra I call home. I have thought hard about every morsel of food before putting it in my mouth. I have stayed away from all possible offenders: all forms of carbs and other unhealthy stuff that made me fat and that I once scarfed down with alarming regularity. I have been a Good Girl and I want—no, I deserve—a standing ovation from everyone in the United States and high fives from the rest of the world. Or at least a pat on the back from *someone*. Is that too much to ask?

Yet nobody—my family, friends, colleagues, *GMA* viewers—says a thing to me about the way I look because the fact is you can't tell I've lost an ounce. *I* can't even tell. Because I am so focused on the number on the scale, on a size and a shape that feels as far away and as impossible as walking to Antarctica, I tell myself that eleven pounds is a drop in the bucket for anyone who needs to lose fifty-plus pounds. It is nothing in the overall scheme. *Nada.*

Instead of celebrating movement in the right direction, I am depressed about what I see as a minuscule weight loss. I worry that Barbara and other ABC News executives are monitoring my progress, or lack thereof, and sharing snide comments about my clear inability or unwillingness to lose weight.

"See, no change. I told you she couldn't do it," I envision thin men in suits saying to Barbara.

There's no way for them to know that I've drastically cut my calorie and carb intake; that I have been on the straight and narrow 24/7 since New Year's Day. That I wake up and spend each and every minute obsessing about *not* eating. That I am constantly hungry and have trouble thinking about *anything* else.

Right now on my bedside table is yet another *People* magazine featuring an "Amazing Weight Loss" cover. In this issue are women who have lost half their size in a year or more.

The old me would have thought it was a waste to spend that much time and effort to reach the goal. No way could I ever stick to that. The truth is that losing anything more than ten pounds in a year—no matter how big you are—is an accomplishment. There is no such thing as catching lightning in a bottle when it comes to weight loss. It takes work.

Yet we have become conditioned to believe that so many things in life are ours for the taking, conveniently ignoring how much time and work is required to accomplish anything significant. Want to get rich? Buy a Powerball ticket. Want to be a superstar? *American Idol* can make you one. *One of the key steps in the Shift is to acknowledge the delusion of quick and easy success.* And to realize once and for all that there is no winning Lotto ticket here. There is no instant gratification, just hard work and patience.

When I think back to all the difficult but worthwhile things I've done in my life—bouncing back from being fired and launching conferences that draw thousands of women each year—none of it was handed to me. Nobody gave me any breaks. I made my own luck and would never have accomplished any of it without sweat and sacrifice. So why haven't I applied that same tenacity to losing weight? Why am I prone to complacency, or, put a less polite way, laziness, when it comes to attacking the dominant issue in my life? Why have I passively waited for something to magically solve this riddle?

The answer is that for most of my adult life, I have denied the obvious: I was not committed. Not truly. I am committed now. For the foreseeable future, that mission will have my undivided attention. I wake up thinking about it, spend my day doing it, and go to bed determined to forge ahead tomorrow. I'm over being fat. This year, I want to look normal and feel good about myself.

And while I'm not thrilled to have lost only eleven pounds, somewhere inside I know that to stay on this journey, to hew to this path, then I have to *celebrate the milestones no matter how tiny they are.*

I can no longer think that "just one" cupcake, piece of bread, or potato chip is acceptable, because the minute I do, I'll slide down that slippery slope to disaster. Temptation is everywhere, and I must learn to deal with it. I can't help but fantasize about a cheat day in my future. If I am really good for two more weeks or another month, maybe then I can look forward to a tasty reward! But as I fantasize about a bowl of cheesy pasta or a soft, warm brownie, I know it's a dangerous idea. Once I have just one treat, I won't stop. I know myself. At this stage, there's no room for moderation or an occasional indulgence. This is basic training and there are no treats.

One of the ways that I make it through these first few months—the hardest period in any kind of Shift—is by finding distractions. I remember a late night in early February when everyone in the house was asleep and I was frustrated with a project that wasn't going as well as planned. I was also exhausted—a dangerous combination for a food addict—and I decided to go to the kitchen to see what kind of possible

snack I could have, even though I knew full well that no
safe snacks were there. I moved my laptop to the side, stood
up from the bed, and walked toward my door. On the edge of
my dresser, I saw a bottle of clear nail polish that Emma had
left there. In a flash, it clicked in my head to grab it, return to
bed, and put on a coat—the first time I had polished my own
nails in years.

I had spent weeks trying to work up a list of good
distractions—take a hot bath or shower, go for a walk—
when I was tempted to cheat. Now, incredibly without looking for it, I had stumbled across a perfect one: you can't do
much of anything with your fingers—like reach deep inside
a bag to grab a handful of chips—until topcoat dries. And it
doesn't dry well for at least a half hour. That night, it proved
long enough to let my hunger pang pass. By the time my nails
had dried I was ready to sleep, and did. Topcoat became my
go-to distraction several more times and probably saved me
thousands of calories and hundreds of carbs that would have
derailed my progress.

Meanwhile, it turns out that my anxiety over not being
noticed was unwarranted. The first email from Barbara
comes this evening, and it's a better reward than any snack.
"You are looking fantastic" is all her note says.

"Aw, so sweet of you to write. Made my day," I respond, as
tears of gratitude well up in my eyes.

8

Avoiding the Doctor, and Failed Diets

Other than going to a walk-in clinic at a Duane Reade drugstore because I was sure I had an ear infection, I have avoided all doctors. The only other recent visit to a doctor was to have precancerous spots removed from my face, which didn't require me to remove my clothing. If it had, I probably would have skipped it. I remember clearly the last time I undressed for a full exam. It was in August 2002—five years after I gave birth to Emma and Jake. I dreaded the thought of going but did it anyway. I was so nervous that day, hoping the doctor wouldn't lecture me about my weight. My blood pressure was slightly elevated, and I quickly made an excuse to the nurse. "White coat hypertension," I said. "Isn't that what it's called when you're terrified to see the doctor?" She smiled and rubbed my shoulder.

My doctor could not have been nicer and spent more than an hour with me on a hot summer afternoon. She knew I was scared: my sweaty palms in the cold, air-conditioned room were a clear giveaway. While going through the thorough exam, she calmed my nerves with a benign conversation about managing kids, motherhood, and career. At the end, she told me she'd step out while I got dressed and that we'd talk again in a few minutes.

I was feeling pretty good, thinking I had dodged the weight bullet. I had made it through the whole exam without being chastised. But then came the final chat. The doctor oh-so-gently recommended that I see her colleague who specialized in obesity.

"He's great," she said, handing me a piece of paper with his name and number. "He'll help you."

I thanked her, but was noncommittal. She made me promise that I wouldn't be a stranger in her office, and I nodded. Of course not. But not only did I *not* follow through on her referral, I also avoided *her* ever since. Just the thought of what I have *not done* for myself in the past decade—no mammogram, pap smear, or blood tests for cholesterol and all the other stuff—now makes my heart race. I'm not proud to admit this—even to myself. I'm filled with shame, especially on behalf of Emma, whom I'd never allow to get to a stage where she is so terrified for any reason, let alone being called fat, that she avoids all doctors. I vowed that I must get a physical—soon. But I wanted to lose more weight first. This is the same story that played out in my mind countless times over the last several years.

So began a series of diets that all seemed to fail me. It wasn't until I made the Shift that I truly understood: *Most diets work, but it's the diet mentality (lose the weight easily and quickly!) that fails us time and again.* And so another walk down memory lane, with all the diets I've tried before.

First, the Cookie Diet. A few years ago, on a family visit to Florida, my mom sheepishly admitted that she was on a new diet.

"I've lost two pounds," she said proudly.

"Fantastic," I said, genuinely happy for her. "How?"

"The Cookie Diet," she said. "My doctor recommended it."

In retrospect, I should have been suspicious. I knew that Mom's doctor was no string bean and was probably desperate—like she and I were—to find a no-pain way of dropping weight. Just because you're an internist doesn't necessarily mean you're not as susceptible as the next person to diet schemes. But I was all ears as Mom explained how the Cookie Diet, invented by Florida weight-loss physician Sanford Siegal, works: you eat nine sixty-calorie cookies during the day to keep hunger away, then a five- to seven-hundred-calorie dinner.

"There are NO failures. Everyone loses weight," Siegal's promotional material promises.

"That's it?" I asked Mom, impressed by its simplicity.

"Yep," she said. "And you know what? It's doable. And the cookies are pretty good."

I eagerly fixated on those two words: "cookies" and "doable." If I had to name a top-five food, cookies would always make the list. And to hear Mom—of all people—say it was "doable," well, where do I sign up?

If she had lost weight on this plan and, more important, said it was *easy*, then it must be a no-brainer. I immediately ordered a three-month supply of cookies and convinced Peter, who wanted to drop some weight, to join me. As the son of a pediatrician, he was impressed that an actual medical doctor developed the cookies and that Mom's internist had endorsed it. At the time, Peter had just left the newspaper business to join me in producing career events for professional women, so it helped if both of us dieted together.

Peter and I ate cookies happily for four days, and although everyone in our office laughed at us, we were pumped: eating cookies during the day wasn't so bad—especially followed by a good meal at night. It all seemed doable, just as promised. But then on the fifth day, I had a lunch date with a colleague that had been scheduled months beforehand.

An old-school type, he invited me to the University Club on Fifty-Fourth Street and Fifth Avenue, where we sat in the vast, mahogany-paneled dining room with its old oil paintings, soaring ceiling, and white linen-covered tables. (Founded in 1865, this is the club that, in 1997, ordered then First Lady Hillary Rodham Clinton to leave after a speech when her lunch companion began talking on a cell phone. That's against club rules and this club doesn't bend its rules for *anyone*.) At various food stations loaded with dozens of choices of appetizers, main courses, and desserts, white-gloved waiters served us whatever we wanted. Lunch for me that day was supposed to be a cookie or two, but there was no way I could escape eating without offending my host. So I indulged. I had to eat lunch, and it all looked too good to pass up, so I went to town. I left the club realizing there was no way I could stay on the Cookie Diet or any extreme plan that demands you stick to one kind of food. I concluded that it was nearly impossible for me to sustain diets like this over the long haul, let alone fit them into real life.

"Fine with me," Peter said when I suggested we abandon the Cookie Diet, eager to dump this latest doozy. That night, we kicked off the weekend with Emma and Jake at Wondee Siam, our favorite Thai restaurant, with spring rolls and basil and curry dishes accompanied by heaping mounds of white rice. Calories and carbs be damned. Full speed ahead.

Months later, I became intrigued hearing about people who had gone on the Zone, which promised to retool your metabolism through an optimal mix of fat, protein, and carbs. I arranged to have Zone meals delivered to my door, and they came like clockwork every morning in an insulated black lunch bag that contained my food for the day. The portions were tasty but small, like what you get on an airplane on a long flight in first class. I was constantly hungry. I managed to lose six pounds in one month, but that wasn't nearly enough for me. I wanted to lose more, *now*. I didn't know it at the time, but impatience consistently undermined every attempt I made to lose weight. Anxious for an even quicker fix, I said so long to the Zone and moved on to the next diet that would, if it really worked, provide faster results.

At this phase, both in terms of dollars and sacrifice, I wanted more bang for my diet buck. Enter the cabbage soup diet, a perennial favorite of celebrities. Supposedly it was initially designed for obese people facing surgery to lose weight fast in the weeks leading up to the procedure for a better surgical outcome. Eat as much cabbage soup as you want, plus specific "reward" foods on each of the seven days you're on it: fruit the first day; then vegetables and a baked potato; beef and tomatoes; and finally brown rice and juices. I found myself voraciously hungry every day for the week I was on the plan, anxiously awaiting whatever the bonus was that night. All for a five-pound weight loss, which, granted, was great for a week's weight loss—but I quickly regained it, as usual, once I went off the plan.

Inevitably, along with millions of others at the time, I had to try the famous Atkins diet. Atkins was actually a breakthrough for me, because I finally got it through my thick, stubborn head that bread, pasta, rice, and basically any food product that is white will make me fat. They are all high in carbohydrates, which our bodies quickly metabolize into sugar, leaving us craving food again a short time later.

But I also found that on Atkins's all-protein diet, I gradually became grossed out by all the meat and fat the plan allowed. Yes, for the first few weeks I loved waking up to the smell of Peter frying thick-sliced, hickory-smoked bacon. And when he'd serve me a classic Atkins-sanctioned breakfast—bacon and eggs scrambled with American cheese—I'd happily gobble it all down. Ditto for the cheeseburger (no bun) with salad for lunch and the steak and creamed spinach at dinner. I had always liked cheese to an extent, but on Atkins I became a connoisseur—or more like a gourmand Cheese Head. Our refrigerator quickly filled with various kinds of Brie, Manchego, and Cheddar. Never mind that cheese is basically all fat—Atkins says it's good for you. Worked for me. But after a short period I felt bloated by saturated fats and desperate for a baked potato, a bag of chips, or a loaf of bread—any freakin' carb I could find. So I quit Atkins, then inhaled carbs for days, quickly erasing whatever strides I had made. Same story, different diet.

Then Peter and I both began David Kirsch's Ultimate New York Body Plan, which calls for a mix of exercise, portion control, low carbs, and lean meat and fish. It was fun doing it with Peter—two motivated people rowing in the same direction—and the plan worked, except Peter started to lose weight much faster than I did. Colleagues quickly noticed he was dropping weight. When we'd walk into our apartment building together, the doormen would comment on his loss—but never mine. I quickly became jealous of his success and began to hammer him relentlessly about how unfair it was. I basically nagged him into quitting and sabotaged our success—all because his loss was greater than mine. I didn't know it at the time, but in any journey like this you'll wait a long time for people to cheer you on, let alone notice what you're up to, because they're too preoccupied with their own issues. I let pettiness and impatience distract me from a plan that was working. Looking back, I'm surprised Peter didn't get angry at me for derailing us both. But he never did. We both lost about eighteen pounds in four months—my greatest victory ever. Until I gained it all back.

In addition to the many diets that I flirted with, my behavior was sometimes outright dangerous. Frustrated by the fact that I couldn't lose weight and keep it off, I turned to StarCaps, diuretics that I took for many months, convinced that I could pee myself thin. Looking back, I have no idea what got into me.

"My father thinks those pills can be problematic," Peter began, gently.

As a physician, his father, Jim, is a credible source, yet in my quest to get thin I rationalized to Peter that my body naturally retains a lot of water, which causes my feet and fingers to swell.

"StarCaps," I explained, "simply allow me to walk comfortably and wear rings without them feeling too tight."

"Dad says diuretics can have serious side effects," Peter pressed, firmer this time.

"Give me a break," I snapped when he gave me a look that said he wasn't really buying it.

He backed off. "I'm sure you know what you're doing, Tory." That ended that discussion.

But I really didn't have a clue. In 2008 StarCaps were pulled from shelves. I panicked because I would no longer have access to a product that I was convinced made me look thinner. I called Mom and begged her to ship me some of her prescription diuretics. I eventually weaned myself from them, because I know they're serious business.

StarCaps weren't the only magic potion I eyed. Maybe if I just took enough QuickTrim pills or powdered drink mixes, I could look just like spokeswoman Kim Kardashian, Emma's hero. I was convinced that KK's genes and willpower—plus her steady stream of trainers, cooks, and assistants—had nothing to do with how fit and beautiful she looked. KK had a trick. They *all* have tricks. If I could only find the one that worked for me!

I cringe now looking at the leftover StarCaps bottle in my medicine cabinet, thinking of the time and money I wasted on snake oil solutions, peddled by those who prey on vulnerable fat women like me. In the past, I tried hard, but my impatience and my circular way of thinking made me give up every time. I drop the StarCaps bottle in the trash where it makes a satisfying thud. No more shortcuts for me.

There's no doubt that all of these diets can lead to weight loss, if followed properly and perhaps indefinitely. But I failed every time because I always gave up too quickly. In retrospect, I know that the worst punishment of that yo-yo insanity has been neglecting routine medical care. *I won't go to the doctor until I lose weight.* It's been ten years since I've had a physical. I'm not about to let another year pass without making an appointment. That stark realization is another powerful motivator to keep me on track.

The Promise of Shapewear

9

have my weekly *GMA* segment in two days and I'm becoming anxious—desperate for a quick fix to accentuate my barely double-digit loss, to show *some* progress. I want my colleagues to notice that I have turned my life around and am not a slacker. I've never been a fan of shapewear—I've always found it too constrictive—but I make an executive decision: I need Spanx. Stat.

"Try to stay positive," Peter says as I head out the door to Bloomingdale's. In the cab ride there, right through Central Park, I think about how I could have walked. It's probably only a mile or so. But it looks like rain and I am tense and, well, no. I notice women of all shapes and sizes in exercise outfits, running, jogging, and speed walking. In a clearing to my left, a close-cropped young man who looks like an army drill sergeant sans uniform is leading a group of eight women through a vigorous series of leg lifts.

I know that at some point I must add exercise to my program, but I ward off that thought as I would the specter of a root canal. *Just don't think about it.* Those high school gym classes are not nearly as distant a memory as they should be: I still have a lingering hatred of exercise. I don't know any weight-loss expert who says you can lose weight and keep it off by simply starving yourself on your couch, remote control in hand. They all say you've not only got to cut back drastically on eating but also burn energy through regular exercise. I'll get there. One thing at a time. But when I arrive at the store, I climb the escalator steps to the fourth-floor lingerie section, instead of just riding up, my tacit nod to exercise. Sort of.

"Hi, hon, can I help you?" asks the friendly salesclerk who stands amid a dizzying display of belly busters, boob lifters, and butt minimizers. I survey the options, my eyes darting around for the magic-sorta-something that will compress my legs. I want something to hide any sight of cottage cheese showing through the lightweight wool pants I plan to wear on TV and to prevent them from rubbing together. The saleswoman, a pretty twentysomething girl with small boobs and a slim waist, says she has just the thing and tries to talk me into what looks like biker shorts. She swears they'll create a super-smooth silhouette under any kind of slacks.

I'm not so sure. I may hate my body, but I know it well. If I buy the size she promises will suck it all in, I envision rolls of flab forming a muffin top above the waistband. I see the same thing inevitably happening at the other end too, creating super-sized doughnuts just above my knees. Why would anyone design leg slimmers that stop mid-thigh instead of extending well below the knee? Am I *really* the only woman whose thigh doesn't miraculously taper and become thin halfway to the knee? This is *so* depressing.

"Go try it on in the dressing room. You'll see," the salesgirl says. She's sweet and means well but is somewhat pushy and aggressive too. Or maybe I'm just anxious and cranky given the circumstances. Undoubtedly the latter.

"No thanks," I say. "I'll just take these," and I place a pile of Spanx on the counter. I'll try them on in my bedroom when I get home, with the door locked. I buy medium control and super control thigh shapers. I also take a "Hide & Sleek" body smoother that looks ridiculously uncomfortable, but I'm hooked on the name. The footless tights are my backup. What they lack in compression, they make up for in comfort. I'm eager to get home and put all of it to the test. When I do, I don't see much difference with the tights, except that it feels awkward to wear pants over the thick nylon/Lycra blend material. One pair of extended panties feels all right, but I'm confused as to why they're not giving me supermodel legs. At best, they've taken an inch off the circumference of the widest part of my thighs. Nobody will notice—because I barely do. *Shit.*

As I stand in front of my bathroom mirror, with less than forty-eight hours before I'm live on-air before millions of viewers, I realize that no matter how much I spend on whatever I buy to hide my shape, these pants I'm wearing are still a size 16. I can't escape looking large. I know on some level that I should be patient with myself. I have been making progress after all, even if it's not yet noticeable. On the other hand, somewhere in the back of my mind, I'm still looking for a way to wiggle out of this predicament. I am convinced that a gimmick exists just for me, that I'll find something that will make me thin, or at least make me *look* thin, like these damn body shapers. Old habits die hard.

I have devoted so much of my life to the Quick Fix, the Shortcut, or the Trick, as opposed to simply—on a daily, consistent basis—eating much less. Instead, I have assiduously latched on to anything or anyone that promised to solve the fat riddle with minimal, if any, discomfort. I've tried every fad diet there is and bought into every weight-loss scheme out there. When it comes to attacking my weight, I morph into a fool. Logic goes out the window.

Have you ever fallen into a routine that just doesn't serve you? It could be the unhealthy lunches, the afternoon sugar fix from the vending machine, the extra cups of coffee that are taking the place of a good night's sleep. You know you want to make a different choice, one that won't feel like deprivation or punishment, but rather will feel *good*. But because almost all change requires work, you stay stuck.

That was me and my Wednesday Chinese takeout dinner the night before my weekly *GMA* segment. Wanted to make a change. Couldn't. Wouldn't. Didn't. For the longest time.

A couple of months into my Shift, I noticed something extraordinary: because that big, unhealthy meal was off the table on Wednesday nights, I no longer woke up early on Thursday mornings feeling so terrible, both emotionally and physically. In fact, the healthier my choices were the night before, the more I practically sprang out of bed when the alarm buzzed. I began to expand the theory further. How else could I tee up my Wednesdays so that I'd feel my best for Thursday's *GMA* spot?

I began a habit of not taking any cabs on Wednesday, which meant I easily logged four or five miles just by walking to and from each place I needed to go. Not enough exercise to drop a size overnight, but it didn't matter. I was discovering that what the Shift had done for my waistline was nothing compared to what it was doing to my confidence. I knew that I was a strong person. Turns out, I was stronger. I knew that no matter what size my clothes were, I was a person of extraordinary focus. You don't juggle a successful business and a career on-air in TV without discipline. But the Shift brought those qualities to the fore. And while the world would eventually get to see the results of the Shift each Thursday when I appeared on *GMA*, it was on Wednesdays that I proved to myself just how committed I could be.

Every woman can do this. Think of a day when the pressure is really on for you. Maybe it's Fridays when you volunteer at your kids' school or have a regular meeting for a charity that you help organize. It could be Monday morning when you have a weekly staff meeting with coworkers who view life as a glass half empty. Perhaps it's Sunday-night dinner with your in-laws or your perennially critical sister and her perfect family. We all have that moment, once a week, many times a week, when we have to show and prove, yet what we really want to do is run and hide. You can use the Shift to bring positive energy to those interactions. The day before, give yourself just a little bit more of what you know makes you feel good—for me, it started with extra exercise and even healthier eating. For others, it may be downloading a ten-minute meditation from iTunes or walking out at lunchtime to splurge on a manicure.

I come to realize that some of the women I admire most— stars like Robin Roberts and Lara Spencer; my *GMA* boss, Margo Baumgart, and executives like Barbara—routinely do this. They shine at work and at home, on- and off-screen, because they are never too busy to consistently make time to do the little and big things that enable them to look and feel their best, especially when the stakes are high. They work at it. This took me years to accept—that *all thin women aren't born that way, nor do they have miraculous metabolisms. They deliberately focus on keeping fit and being at the top of their game because it matters.*

That Thursday morning, I shimmied into the Spanx for

my *GMA* segment, hoping that if the big bosses were watching, they would see that I was smaller than I was three months ago, that I have made progress, and that I am with the program. The shapewear didn't shave pounds off, but it did smooth out my still substantial curves. I was eating right. I was walking. I may not have been slimming down as fast as I wanted to, but I will give myself credit for sticking to the Shift. This was going through my head as J.C., the audio guy, clipped the battery pack to the back of my pants, ran the wired microphone up the front of my blouse, then gently whispered, "Hey, you're losing weight. Good for you." I don't know if it was the shapewear or the confidence I felt from being true to my Shift the day before, but when the camera went live, I was beaming.

make the *Shift*

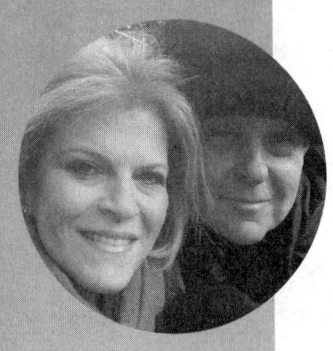

Most diets work, but it's the diet mentality (lose the weight easily and quickly!) that fails us time and again.

What the Shift will do for your waistline is nothing compared to what it will do for your confidence and self-esteem. Give yourself credit for each healthy meal and for every mile walked.

MONTH 4

10

Hope Is Not a Strategy

My friend Heidi Krupp and I are having a long-awaited lunch at Gabriel's, a media hangout on the Upper West Side a few doors down from the apartment where Peter and I first lived after we were married. Heidi is running a bit late, and I'm recalling the baby shower my friends gave me here fourteen years earlier when I was pregnant with Emma and Jake. It was the very definition of a power shower. Bringing two babies into the world at once at age twenty-six . . . talk about a shift!

Heidi arrives and says she's starving. Her baby boy has kept her up half the night, she overslept, and, well, let's eat! A special on this spring day is pappardelle with mushrooms in truffle oil with a light dusting of Parmigiano-Reggiano cheese. It's the kind of dish that sends me into food heaven because I love all four ingredients.

"Oh my gosh, imagine that," Heidi says. "Sooo bad."

Of course I want the pasta special. Desperately. I can taste those rich, buttery flat noodles covered in *funghi*. The aroma in Gabriel's is out of control, and the waiter has placed a bread basket between us, pouring a dollop of green virgin olive oil into a small plate for dipping. *Go ahead, little piggies, eat.* But I don't. I've already perused the menu and found a healthier option, one that has become a mainstay for me in the last three months: chicken paillard—a thinly pounded breast, grilled and topped with fresh arugula.

"Boy, you really *are* being good," Heidi says, as she orders the same dish.

"Damn right," I say, looking her in the eyes with a smile.

At lunch, Heidi and I talk about everything except how I am doing weight-wise, but as we walk out, she can't contain herself any longer.

"So how's it going?" she asks, gesturing to my body.

"Ha! Just spit it out," I say, because I know what she's really asking. "How much weight have I lost? Is that what you're getting at?"

"I was trying to be subtle!" She laughs.

"Only seventeen pounds, which is a lot less than I originally thought I would've lost by now," I tell her. "When I lost nine pounds in the first three weeks, I thought I'd just continue on that path. Three pounds a week sounded so reasonable, which meant I'd be down thirty now. But by the end of March, I had lost a little more than fifteen pounds and knew then that three pounds a week was unrealistic. So I stopped putting a number on it. I know now that this is going to take time."

"You're the most impatient person I know," Heidi says. "How painful is it for you to be good?"

"It's a conscious effort. I'm constantly thinking about eating and not eating," I tell her. "Has it gotten easier? Yes. But is it a breeze? Definitely not. I am very eager to get to twenty pounds lost."

"You're almost there! I love your guts," Heidi says, as we hug good-bye.

Heidi knows me well. The truth is that I *am* impatient. Once I committed to a plan that had slow and steady weight loss at the core, I needed to fuel my Shift with inspiration. It's easy to feel lousy when the scale hasn't moved for days or weeks, even though I was making smart choices for every meal. During those frustrating times, I would make collages. Old-fashioned collages. I curled up on the couch with a stack of magazines and I'd cut out words that reflected how I wanted the world to see me—*confident, poised, satisfied, loyal, curious, happy, generous, extraordinary,* among others. I brushed decoupage glue on top of each word and placed it face-up on the bottom of a clear glass plate that I purchased at a nearby craft store, until words filled the surface. Each time, these three-hour projects were a great distraction from snacking on lazy weekend afternoons. And the result empowered me: I had a beautiful one-of-a-kind piece of art and the whole process was soothing and enjoyable. Moreover, each day, I had all of these inspiring words and images to encourage me.

The Take-Out Girls

11

One morning, I'm just out of the shower when Peter asks, "Turkey bacon and eggs?"

"No, thanks, I'm not hungry."

I know that every diet guru says to start your day with a good breakfast. As such, whenever I tried to lose weight before, that's what I did. But the Shift is a lifestyle reboot—not strictly a diet—and part of it includes coming up with guidelines that work for *me*, even if they're unconventional from a diet standpoint. Instead of getting nowhere with other plans, this is about charting a new course that gets results *for me*.

The truth is I rarely wake up starving. When my mind is

engaged—reading a newspaper, watching *GMA*, seeing my kids off to school, showering and getting to work—I rarely think about food. Most days I can easily skip breakfast and make it to lunch without it affecting me at all. The clock will not set my eating choices: If I am not hungry, I won't eat. That makes me feel good because the more calories I save with little stunts like this, the faster I will lose weight.

But lunch in my office is trickier. I work with a staff of six—five women, plus Peter—planning events for professional women. Our office is one open space on the fourth floor of a busy block on the Upper West Side. It takes an intensive marketing and sales effort to reach attendees and sponsors, which we do online and on the phone. This is also where calls come in and packages arrive throughout the day for my *GMA* segments. I often refer to it as organized chaos. None of us has a cubicle, let alone a private office, which means that when anyone eats something it's obvious to all of us. Similarly, when one person starts talking about food, it's usually just a matter of minutes before others chime in.

"I'm thinking chicken fingers," our sales manager says halfway through the morning.

"Pizza," her junior associate chimes in, not looking up from her desktop.

I look at the clock. It's only 10:30, a little early to be thinking about lunch, isn't it? And yet at one point I would have been right there with them, eagerly planning my next food fix. For more than a decade, my most senior employee has led the charge Monday to Friday, rattling off menu options before she's finished her coffee. When her favorite coworker joined us years later, it's as if they'd found kindred spirits: two foodies who spend part of every day figuring out what goodies they'll eat next. Pizza from Ray's. Gyro platters from the Greek Kitchen. A BLT from the Broadway Diner. Chicken fingers from Big Nick's. Then for an afternoon snack they fantasize about the daily flavors of frozen yogurt at the place across the street, or perhaps a few cupcakes from the shop just a few doors east of us. Most days, it's barely noon and white Styrofoam platters dot our desks, the smell of fatty, greasy food palpable as you walk off the elevator toward our office. Once I make the Shift, the temptation to join them—which I did more times than not over the years—is excruciating until I find my groove on my new plan.

My commitment to avoiding the lunchtime fast-food binges forces me to look for and stick to healthier choices. I cling to a safe bet: a salad from a little restaurant five blocks from our office called Chirping Chicken. It's famous not just for its grilled chicken but because the daughter of the owner won half of a $45 million New York Lotto some years ago.

Chirping's Greek salad is delicious—piled high with grilled chicken, a few slices of tomatoes, two black olives, a stuffed grape leaf, a hot pepper, and a few carrot shreds. I savor the olives and trade Peter my grape leaf and hot peppers for his two olives when we both order the salad. Sometimes I hit the Chirping jackpot and they accidentally give me three of the little suckers. When I need a change of pace, I walk a block and pick up a grilled chicken Cobb salad from Le Pain Quotidien, but I swap the blue cheese, which I don't like, for

Parmesan, which I love. The salad is a satisfying mix of bits of bacon, fresh avocado, diced tomato, and bite-sized pieces of white meat chicken, with a light splash of vinaigrette. The to-go size is much smaller than the restaurant serving—a small box verses a large plate. That annoyed me at first, but I came to appreciate that built-in portion control is a good thing.

While I stick to salads for lunch, late-afternoon snack cravings usually kick in and are harder to deal with. Snacks are dicey—they add up—especially when others in the office routinely reach for them. Alex, who plans our events, often announces she is going on a froyo run—who's in? I hired her two years ago right out of the University of Michigan and am impressed with what a fast learner and consummate professional she is. Alex and I have had some interesting chats about food and weight loss. She's got a perfect little figure herself but is not obsessed with being über thin, a by-product of a scary bout with anorexia in college. She is acutely aware of the tricky balance between being thin but not over the top. Her mission now, she has told me, is just to be healthy and eat in moderation, which includes an afternoon treat.

Of course I want to join her, but I say no. When the thought of sitting at my desk watching her eat spoonfuls of Pinkberry frozen yogurt is too much, I use a little trick that I've come to rely on: I get up and take a walk around the block. For years, I never moved from my desk between lunch and when I left for the day. Now I frequently take a fifteen- or twenty-minute walk in the neighborhood and find that just getting up and moving gives me the same little afternoon boost that an Oreos bender would have before. Some days, if the craving for something sweet is particularly strong, I go to Starbucks or Aroma, a popular coffee shop three doors away, for an iced coffee or a small cappuccino. Like Target lemonade, a cappuccino is relatively guilt-free for me.

I am particular (Peter might say demanding and unreasonable) about how I like my cappuccino: super dry, which in coffee shop parlance means espresso with plenty of foam but not a lot of milk, because too much milk adds too many carbs. Sometimes this makes me the Starbucks Customer from Hell. A Barista's Worst Nightmare. The Cappuccino Witch whose photo they throw darts at during breaks in the back room. I feel badly about that, really, I do, but I'm a stickler on this since I don't like drinking my carbs—I'd rather eat them. It's java joy for me when I place my order and the server instantly knows what I'm talking about. While I usually sprinkled a Sweet'N Low into my steaming cappuccino, I discover that a little cinnamon on top is a tasty and healthier alternative.

More often than not, when I return to my desk the cravings are gone. But today I come back to find a package from Cheryl's Cookies filled with three dozen individually wrapped cookies—chocolate chip, chocolate chocolate chip, peanut butter, and sugar. The company has sent this in hopes of landing a spot in my *GMA* segment. But as the smell of butter and chocolate wafts through the air, I shut the box and pass it to my colleagues, who are only too happy to dive in for a sweet treat. It's a work hazard that I am around food all the time, and I know I've got to resist these near-constant temptations. Just one of Cheryl's undoubtedly delicious cookies would account for my entire daily carb allotment. And I know myself: I wouldn't stop at just one, which means my mindless snack would have an excellent chance of killing my entire week.

As the girls sample each type of cookie, I keep telling myself that the *momentary* pleasure I'd get from binging on sweets isn't worth the pain of seeing the needle move to the right on the scale. I can't bear the agony of knowing that I have let myself down—again. But what finally gets me through the afternoon is knowing that for the past few days, I have been creeping up on my next milestone. I think tonight may be the moment I reach it, and I won't be waylaid by a chocolate chip cookie. So I dive back into work, content that I have resisted temptation.

"Let's go," Peter says to me just after 6 P.M. "I want to pick up some things on the way home."

"Like my pickles?"

"Absolutely," he says.

I've become addicted to pickles, which have become my go-to, predinner snack. Not just any pickles: I insist on Ba-Tampte ("MEANS TASTY," says the label) kosher pickles. The serving size on the label is preposterous: one-third of a pickle, as if anyone would eat only that portion. But that serving has zero calories, zero fat, and less than one carb, which means a whole pickle is a safe snack. I only need one of these crunchy, briny, garlicky things to satisfy me—odd, since I don't like cucumbers, which is a shame since they're so Shift-worthy.

Back in January, my hunger pangs were in high gear, and my suddenly reduced calorie intake was making me sorta bitchy. One rainy night we had a pickle predicament when I realized we were fresh out of them, and I was desperate for a fix.

"What are you going to do about this?" I asked Peter not too nicely, as he was about to sit down to watch *Dexter.* He glared at me.

"Dad and I will walk Marly and check out every supermarket within a twenty-block radius until we find your pickles," Jake sweetly piped up. No way he wanted to have Bad Mood Mom around all night.

My boys ended up on an hour-long scavenger hunt to seven supermarkets and a dozen bodegas that probably serve a million New Yorkers within a one-mile radius of our apartment. But no luck. Jake later admitted to me that he was worried about returning home empty-handed and having to tell the Picky Pickle Princess that they failed in their mission. Peter was more comfortable with it, and all he said at the time was "No dice. Sorry, babe." Yet since then, I notice Peter has made sure we always have at least two jars of my brand in the refrigerator at all times.

When I reflect on that night, and how demanding I was of Peter and Jake, I cringe. But the truth is that severely cutting back on any longtime habit often makes people moody. At least it did with me at first. In my defense, I wasn't myself because I had completely upended the rhythm of my life and it affected my mood. I pledged early on that I wouldn't force my food choices on my family. Now I have to remind myself that cutting back on calories and carbs can make me irritable. Peter told me that when he quit smoking he feared he wouldn't be able to write a word of his column without a cigarette and wouldn't be any fun to be around, so he took a week off from work. He spent every day using a handsaw to take down several trees, which he then cut into small pieces. I'm not into sharp objects, but I distract myself from thinking about food when I can, and I'm learning to be patient with myself in terms of occasional mood swings. Sometimes simply taking a few deep breaths is what keeps me from snapping.

make the *Shift*

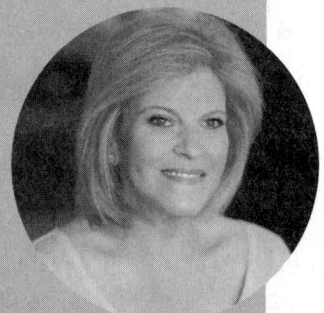

Stop putting a number on your weekly goal. Trust that this will take time.

Let an afternoon walk around the block take the place of your afternoon snack.

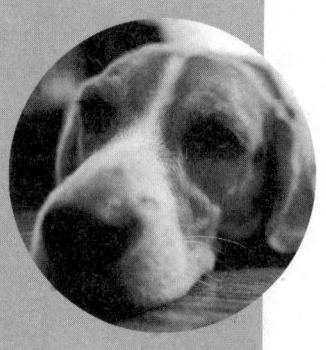

MONTH 5

12

Kiss the Chef!

onight's stop at Fairway is a rarity for me. The always jam-packed supermarket is an Upper West Side institution, and this evening is no exception, with busy professionals, young moms wielding strollers, and two people on a healthy-eating mission packing the store's narrow aisles. Peter loves grocery shopping, so I'm happy to leave it to him; it also spares me from being surrounded by temptation.

"Eighteen dollars a pound?" Peter asks at the seafood counter, eyeing me as if I am insane to want fresh fillet of sole.

"Look at the money we're saving by me skipping all the junk I used to eat," I say with a smile.

97

"Which has been offset by all those *dry* cappuccinos," he teases, not letting me have the last word.

Later, when I walk in the kitchen, he's proud of the fish he's just cooked, which has filled the air with a lemony garlic scent that smells great, as does the green kale he's serving with it. I used to hate the taste of kale—too bitter—but it became one of my favorites once Peter sautéed it in a bit of olive oil with a few scallions, chopped red bell pepper, and diced turkey bacon.

Lean proteins are now my main meals of choice, which means we eat a lot of chicken breasts as well as shrimp, flounder, salmon, and sole. A couple times a month I'll have breakfast for dinner: scrambled eggs with bits of smoked salmon or eggs scrambled with mushrooms and some sort of cheese. We all love steaks but they're fatty, so we limit red meat to once every few weeks.

Since a girl can't live on arugula, iceberg, and romaine alone, I go for vegetables I like that are lowest in carbs. Broccoli, cauliflower, mushrooms, asparagus, artichokes, celery, and tomatoes become my go-to options. Off-limits for me are the higher-carb choices like corn, carrots, and beans.

Peter experiments regularly with different spices, and I find that curry, sage, dill, rosemary, and garlic do wonders for sauces and marinades. Also a half cup of chicken broth poured over sautéing vegetables and then covered quickly creates a tasty steam-cooked flavor. In pre-Shift days, we would invariably have some sort of pasta, rice, or potato with each meal, but I cleared our cabinets of that stuff, and for the most part it has been out of sight, out of mind for all of us. No one seems to cry for it, but they do miss other food groups.

"Can't we ever have ice cream around here?" Jake pleaded one night, fed up with the lack of junk food in our kitchen. "Would it kill us to have some normal food in this house?"

"Mom doesn't want that stuff around because she'll be tempted to eat it. Can you blame her?" Peter asked.

"No," Jake said, somewhat annoyed. "But just because she's on a diet doesn't mean I have to be."

"Good point," Peter told him, and later took me aside to relay Jake's frustration. Clearly I had violated my own resolution to not impose food choices on my family. Peter said he knew very well why I didn't want to have snacks staring me in the face every time I walked into the kitchen. He understood that eating healthy food and teaching our kids the value of good nutrition was one thing. But to keep two growing teenagers from occasionally indulging in some junk food wasn't fair to them. He was right. That day, for the first time in months, Jake and Emma walked to the store with Peter and selected ice cream, popcorn, chips, and salsa. A week later, a lot of it was untouched, which proves they both have healthy eating habits. Early on, I would have felt tortured at having junk food in the house, but now it's not as bad as I thought. This was a first for me, a point of pride to no longer find myself locked in a dire mental struggle when it came to tempting food. I could smell Ruffles or Cheez-Its and not go into a panic mode or frenzy like our beagle, Marly, does around anything edible. The Shift was working.

As Peter takes out dinner plates and begins to serve us the sole, I see a small bag of Fritos that Jake has left on the counter—the type of snack that I once ate routinely without even thinking. I read the label. The serving size is just one ounce, with 160 calories and 15 carbs. But this bag contains *three* servings—and I can't ever recall *not* eating the whole thing. So that's 480 calories and a stunning 45 carbs in that tiny bag. I'm shocked that I used to eat foods like this, with so little regard to these numbers. Which is exactly why I have become obsessed with reading nutrition labels, something I purposely avoided because I didn't want proof of how poorly I was eating.

Now I know that "low fat" often means "high sugar," which means out of the question for me, and that often a food will at first glance appear to be low carb, until the serving size reveals it's only so when you eat a smidgen—something no one ever does. Like this six-ounce bag of Price Chopper brand Crispy Onions from our cabinet. It's a version of those tasty french-fried rings you sprinkle on the top of string bean casseroles. Only four carbs per serving. Not bad! Then I see that a serving size is one and a half *teaspoons*—roughly enough to satisfy a hunger pang of a field mouse—and this six-ounce pack has *twenty-four* servings. That's ninety-six carbs in one little pack or my carb limit for *four* days.

(I am grateful to New York mayor Michael Bloomberg,

who pushed a law that requires many restaurants in the city to display the calorie counts of menu items. It's forced me to pay more attention to food choices and I don't see any downside to that. At the very least we can't claim ignorance when we order reduced-fat banana chocolate chip coffee cake at Starbucks and discover it contains a whopping four hundred calories and eighty carbs.)

I toss the crispy critters in the trash and call the kids to dinner, where we dive into yet another delicious meal. Peter loves to cook, prepares all our meals, and rarely gets any complaints from us no matter what he serves. I don't know if my Shift would be as seamless without his contributions in the kitchen.

13

Twenty Pounds Down

Later that night, it's time to face the scale. To keep myself motivated and not tempted to cheat, I weigh myself every day. Normal fluctuations in weight might drive some people crazy, but they keep me on track. If I'm up, it toughens my resolve. If I'm down, I become more determined to soldier on. With rare exception, I weigh myself when I wake up, but tonight I hop on the scale because I am hoping I have reached a milestone. I'm too impatient to wait until morning, even though I realize there's a danger in weighing myself after dinner when I'm feeling full. But when the needle on the scale settles into three digits, I know I did it. I lost twenty pounds—the most weight I have shed in my life. You might think I would be over the moon about this. But my emotions are mixed: it's terrific news, there's no denying that, but as I stand in front of the mirror, whatever high I feel is deflated by knowing that I have so far to go. In the scheme of things, what I've done is just a small step in a very long road ahead.

Still, the numbers on the scale prove my plan is working. If I ever worried about being too rigid, the results put that fear to rest. Always thinking ahead, deliberately focusing on what's acceptable and what's not, and sticking to it has worked so far. As has become a habit, I mentally review all my tried-and-true guidelines:

- Limit carbs to under twenty-five per day. I have gotten to know carb counts by religiously reading nutrition labels or looking them up online before eating.
- Cut portions by eating half or less of my pre-Shift serving sizes.
- Stick to proteins such as lean meats (chicken, fish), eggs, and limited cheese.
- Eat low-carb fresh vegetables, including lettuce varieties, broccoli, cauliflower, mushrooms, asparagus, artichokes, celery, and tomatoes.
- Skip starchy vegetables that are high in carbs, such as carrots, corn, and beans.
- Avoid all fruit, juices, and smoothies. (When I reach at least a thirty-pound weight loss, I will add fresh berries from time to time.)

- Absolutely no soda, including diet.
- Nothing white: potatoes, pasta, rice, bread, flour, and sugar are off-limits. To be even more specific, no candy, cake, cupcakes, cookies, or related stuff. Skip the sugar-free varieties as well.
- Know that "low-fat" and "reduced-fat" packaged foods often mean "high sugar," which make them no-nos.
- Steer clear of fast food, pizza joints, bakeries, and candy stores. Cook at home and make eating out or ordering in the exception.
- When tempted to try something bad, pause for a few minutes and look for a distraction before giving in. Avoid situations where it may be too painful or difficult to *not* cheat.
- Replace food treats and rewards with inedible ones, like a manicure, a ten-minute massage, or fresh flowers.
- Weigh myself daily.
- If I should slip, start over instantly, without delay. Any moment can be Day One if necessary.

Five months in, what started as a minute-by-minute struggle—always wondering when I could eat next—is still top of my mind, but it's no longer the epic battle that it was in January. It's just my reality. Perhaps my experience as a small business owner is helping me with this process. When I have a financial goal, I don't simply try hard and hope for the best. I create a plan—not some cumbersome forty-page document that leaves me exhausted by the end. Just something clear and concise with step-by-step instructions on how I expect to make it happen. I reserve the right to adjust as needed along the way, but abandoning the goal is never an option, especially one where money is involved. That's how I am approaching this: *My mission is getting to a healthy weight, and I can alter my plan if necessary, but I'll never bail on the process.*

Eating much less becomes a point of private pride. I don't walk around saying, "Look how little I put down my gullet today." But as a woman who used to mindlessly snack and eat with abandon, consciously *not eating* is new and exciting. Like a ballet dancer who happily chomps away at her celery sticks because she is dancing for the company of her dreams, I realize that there is freedom in the discipline I've imposed on myself. *I am not punishing myself as I thought early on in the Shift. I am making choices, and every time I exert a healthy choice, I remind myself that I am free to be a different person from the one I was my whole life.* Julie Andrews once said, *"Some people regard discipline as a chore. For me, it is a kind of order that sets me free to fly."* I am not flying yet, but there are days when I think of how much weight I've lost and how good I feel, and my feet barely touch the ground.

The Skinny Girls' Secret

14

"What's your secret?" Cindy asks. "Come on, tell me what you're doing."

Cindy and I are in my room at the Marriott near Pike Place Market in Seattle. It's late and she's traveling with me for Spark & Hustle, my nationwide series of small business conferences. I adore Cindy. She's smart and ebullient—and wears her heart on her sleeve. A blond, brown-eyed former Miss Oklahoma contestant (third runner-up!), she loves to flutter her long fake eyelashes.

For years, she was a well-known local Tulsa TV anchor until, at age forty-three, a very public firing ended her career—one, she tells our audiences, she expected would have lasted well into her third face-lift. That always gets a laugh. Within months, the shame of being let go in a city where everyone knew her name, coupled with a health scare, conspired to add thirty-five pounds on the frame of a five-foot-six-inch gal who once strode confidently on stage in heels and a bathing suit. That she is overweight bugs this beauty enormously, enough so that she's been on and off Weight Watchers with inconsistent results. Cindy has told me many times that she'd like to lose forty-five pounds—more than our beagle weighs, as Emma pointed out to me a couple years ago when I said I wanted to lose that much. "That's more than Marly weighs, Mommy!"

Cindy and I met online when she read that I said good-bye to corporate America and started my own business after I was fired from NBC News. We became friends bonding via email over job-loss and eventually over our weight-loss struggles too. Cindy has sat next to me from morning to night at a dozen daylong conferences and she's noticed things are very different these days. Not only in the way I am physically shrinking, albeit slowly, but also that I sometimes skip lunch and no longer engage in mindless consumption, which she and I always used to do together just a year earlier. She has picked up that I no longer touch any of the York Peppermint Patties, Andes mints, or Hershey's Kisses that we put on every table as a little pick-me-up for our attendees. A Diet Dr Pepper addict, she has noticed—and mentioned to me—how I'm no longer drinking Diet Pepsi. "What's up with the water?" she scribbled on a piece of paper during one New York event, as Barbara Corcoran of *Shark Tank* got some laughs from the stage.

Now she's sitting on my hotel bed in sweatpants, picking at fresh chocolate chip cookies that an Oregon woman who is starting a baked goods business has given me, hoping I'll like them and feature her products on TV. Cindy eyes the bottle of wine that a banquet manager has left as a thank-you for hosting the event and asks if it's okay to open it.

"Of course," I say. "Go for it."

There are no wineglasses, so Cindy takes one of the short, faux crystal cups from the bathroom and fills it with Chardonnay.

"Come on," she says conspiratorially, taking a sip. "You look great. Tell me what's going on. I need your secret."

I can relate to Cindy's eagerness for answers, but I suspect she'll be disappointed to learn that I have no big secret, only a lot of discipline and hard work. Before I answer her, I ask how badly she wants to lose weight. She rattles off a series of adverbs: "hugely," "desperately," "majorly." She seems serious, but as much as I love her, I'm skeptical. I know Cindy. Living with her on the road, I've watched her eating and drinking habits for months now and I doubt she's ready to make the Shift. So I start with what I view as an easy, obvious question.

"Are you willing to give up drinking?"

Ouch. I can see the shock in her face. "You mean stop having wine?" she asks, holding up her now half-empty glass, mid-toast.

I nod. That's exactly what I mean.

"Nah, I don't think I can go without my white wine at night or my margaritas with girlfriends," she replies without pausing to ponder the question.

"Then you're not serious about losing weight," I say dismissively. So much for her being hugely, desperately, and majorly serious.

I see the hurt on Cindy's face. She was not prepared for the question and I immediately regret how blunt I was. I came on way too strong. But I couldn't help myself when all I can think of is how many times I walked in her shoes, desperate to lose those forty-five pounds but basically indifferent—numb, in fact—to the sacrifice it would take to do it. How until this year I had never considered that I'd have to put *anything and everything* on the line—all the goodies I had enjoyed my entire life—to make the Shift. In Cindy's case, this is not about me being anti-alcohol—I have nothing against people who enjoy wine, beer, or spirits—it's about her unwillingness to put *everything* edible on the table and up for grabs. Until I embraced that concept—really wrapped my head around it—I was always doomed to fail.

I know that in Cindy's case, a daily glass or two of wine or fruity cocktails on a girls' night out won't cut it if she's serious about reincarnating herself as a fortysomething beauty queen. The biggest difference between Cindy and me right now is our state of mind. You can't begin this journey until you're ready—really ready, not half-assed ready—and I recognize some of the same fear and hesitancy in her that I felt before the Shift. Significant change is daunting, but doing it often comes down to preference or priority. My *preference*—hands down—is to eat whatever I want, whenever I want; just like Cindy wants to be able to have her wine or cocktails every night. But my *priority* is to lose a lot of weight, which means it must always trump my cravings and food preference. *When it comes down to it, the question is: What is your priority and what are you willing to forgo to achieve it?*

A few days later, I am doing my weekly live segment on the number one local news station in the country, New York's WABC, where I am promoting a decidedly *un-diet* cookie. In my segments, just as I do on *Good Morning America*, I feature exclusive deals on an array of products from local businesses, everything from food items to cookware to clothing and accessories. I am welcomed by three pencil-thin anchors—Liz Cho, a talented beauty with long dark hair and chiseled features; David Novarro, her gracious on-air partner; and meteorologist Lee Goldberg, whom I tease on-air relentlessly and have arbitrarily picked as my little Mikey, the kid from the Life cereal commercials from my youth. I start every segment with a food product and use Lee as my guinea pig. He plays along, always eager to taste it. *He likes it! He likes it!* And the camera pans to him as he vigorously samples the cookies, s'mores, truffles, chocolate-covered pretzels, cupcakes, and kettle corn that I put in front of him.

But I notice that while Lee and his two colleagues *taste* what I have brought on-air to play along, they rarely *finish* a cookie or devour candy when we break for a commercial and viewers are no longer there to watch. I've been around on-air TV people for more than twenty years, and yet it only finally dawns on me: *that's why they're all so thin.*

Preference or priority. I can't help but believe that most TV news anchors would *prefer* to gobble all those sugary treats just as their off-air colleagues do when I hand out all the leftovers from my segments. But, the anchors know that TV is a visual medium and viewers like to see fit people on-air, so their *priority* becomes staying trim and keeping their jobs. *Duh.* Sacrificing what they'd *like* to do with what they *have* to do looms large in their lives. Now it does in mine too, not just because of my three minutes on national and local TV each week, but because I am so determined to not spend the rest of my life as a fatty.

While the anchors at WABC have mastered the ability to take just a bite, until I can prove that I can lose much more weight, I'm not allowing myself to go there. It takes an almost religious commitment since there are constant opportunities each and every day, but my guidelines keep me on track. Yes, *my willpower is constantly tested, but I find it's like a muscle: the more I use it the stronger it becomes.* Whenever I dieted before, I imagined that I would suffer acute desperation and craving day in and day out. That made the whole endeavor so discouraging. Who wants to feel like that, like they are in prison, trapped by an unyielding diet?

But now I realize that while the beginning was hard, with time it got much easier. That happened after about six weeks, in early February as Valentine's Day approached.

For years, the holiday was an excuse to eat all things chocolate, especially gigantic chocolate-covered strawberries that Peter would buy for me at the Godiva store a block from our office. While he was there he'd also pick up a dozen or so truffles for an extra love treat. But this time around, he knew that this stuff was off-limits. So he bought me a large bouquet of pink roses instead with a note that said, "I love you. Don't eat these!" As I was admiring them, the FedEx guy walked into our office with three boxes containing an assortment of—you guessed it—chocolate-covered strawberries from Shari's Berries, another potential *GMA* segment offering. In the past there would have been no question: I would have eaten two, three, or maybe five of those hunks of fruity chocolate. But this time, I would resist temptation because I was in a different place. Why spoil a good thing? Did I wish I could eat them? Of course. Would it hurt to indulge just a little? Maybe not. Still, I said no because I was not ready to test whether I could be satisfied with just one. I know my limits. When Easter came along several weeks later, I wasn't even slightly tempted to buy bags of crunchy, candy-coated mini Cadbury eggs, something I had done without fail for years.

I imagine it must be similar to addicts getting past withdrawal. In the throes of it, you can't fathom living another second without a hit, but once the urgency passes, the long haul becomes more manageable. There's peace on the other side. Now five months into the Shift, I feel pretty strong. Stronger than I would have predicted.

That night, after I get home, my iPhone pings and it's an email from Barbara. "You are looking great. Hope you're feeling well. Let's do another breakfast or lunch soon." What a difference a few months can make. Another breakfast—as if the first one wasn't enough! Gotta love Barbara, and the truth is I'm thrilled that she's noticing, because she set me on this journey that has already given me so much.

make the Shift

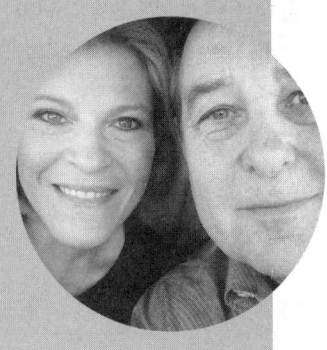

I am not punishing myself. I am making choices. For every healthy one, I am free to be a different person from who I was in the past.

Remember the Julie Andrews quote: "Some people regard discipline as a chore. For me, it is a kind of order that sets me free to fly."

MONTH 6

The Saboteur

arbara's email fuels me to keep going and reminds me that all the sacrifices I am making are worth it. But not everyone understands or accepts my level of commitment. My friend Scott is tall, just an inch shy of six feet, with a smile that disarms the moment you meet him. He's a sports fanatic, but he's also crazy about all things food: Food Network, grilling, trying new recipes, scanning menus online, grocery shopping, you name it. He and I met a few years ago when he ran a live web chat about job searching at an unemployment office in the Bronx. We got to know each other in and out of work, and he's now a close friend.

His lack of acceptance of my Shift became clear when I

asked him to help me scout a few locations in Atlanta for my
Spark & Hustle conference. Since Peter was tied up and had
to stay in New York, he suggested that Scott join me for the
day. After a busy Sunday checking out venues, we sit down
at a restaurant to eat a late afternoon lunch. Neither of us
has eaten all day. But only one of us is moody—and it's not
me. Scott orders a sushi appetizer and Parmesan-crusted scal-
lops accompanied by lobster risotto. I get a chopped salad appetizer and three pieces of spicy tuna sashimi. As Scott digs
into his seafood, I slowly nibble at my plate. Suddenly, he goes
on the offensive.

"There's no way you're not going to eat all of that," he
says.

"I'm eating," I protest, essentially telling him to chill. But
what I'm really doing is picking. I've become an expert
picker, especially in social settings—moving pieces around
the plate and from side to side instead of shoveling food into
my mouth. I routinely leave food on my plate, which is what
I've noticed so many healthy people do—only they get away
with it, without attracting any notice or fuss. I'm not there
yet. Or at least as far as my buddy Scott is concerned.

"I'm calling Peter!" he says. "This is ridiculous. Not eating
is no way to lose weight."

I'm tempted to laugh—*uh, that's exactly how you lose
weight*—until I realize that he's serious and actually quite
worked up about it. I know why: he has watched a few friends
and relatives take diets to the extreme, and they've gotten
sick by doing so. His diet theory is that eating reasonable

portions of whatever you'd like is the way to eventually lose and ultimately settle into a normal weight. Possibly true, but I've never been disciplined enough to eat *reasonable* portions of anything I want, which is why I'm fat. But instead of getting into a fight, I smile because I know Scott means well and there's no winning this argument. I also know that I'm right, at least when it comes to my personal approach, and the scale in my bathroom backs me up.

On the flight back to New York, I think about how I used to eat: until I was stuffed. I'd wipe my plate clean, like a Depression-era child who was not sure when her next meal might come. Or a fat Miami Beach kid who just got in the habit of gorging herself. Now I eat until I'm satisfied, or until I think it's enough. *Big* difference.

Earlier this summer, Scott spent the weekend at our house in the country with Peter and me while his wife and son were out of town. For dinner, Peter grilled steak and some peppers, onions, and zucchini, which he served with a tossed salad. We ate as the sun faded on the patio by our pool.

"Hey, let's go to Twin Cone," Peter suggested, prompting the three of us to hop into the Honda and head down Mountain Road toward Route 17.

Twin Cone, a drive-in ice-cream shop with long lines, huge selections, and a near-mythological local reputation, takes its name from the two giant ice-cream-cone-shaped billboards on its roof. For fifteen summers, I rarely missed a single weekend when I didn't order a lemon ice, soft-serve chocolate with chocolate sprinkles, or a mint chocolate mixer with brownie bits. It was a routine sugar fix.

On this night, Peter had a cone with two large scoops of strawberry and chocolate ice cream. Scott went for chocolate chip on a wafer cone. I passed, happily. Twin Cone was off-limits.

About an hour later, when we returned from Peter's tour of the town, we took out the Scrabble board. I found it was missing a few tiles. There's a mall in nearby Middletown, and Scott suggested we go buy a new set. Peter had no intention of going since he hates the game and had been looking forward to getting to Daniel Silva's latest spy thriller, *The Fallen Angel*, which he'd picked up that day. Out of nowhere, Scott seemed like he was in a sullen mood. Uh-oh. I found it hard to believe a few lost Scrabble pieces would set him off. But in the car I quickly learned what was bugging him.

"Your eating habits are insane," he seethed when we headed back down the mountain. "You didn't touch more than a few bites of steak. And who skips the chance to have even a small ice cream?"

Clearly he was worked up about this—again—only this time instead of just smiling I cut him off. I wasn't amused and I didn't want to take any more of his nonsense.

"Shut up," I blurted out at him, angry. "Do I look like a girl who's sick or starving? Give me a break."

When we got to Target, I let him buy us a new game. On the way back home he explained again that he'd seen too many people close to him lose too much weight too fast.

"It can get out of control," he said. "You should watch it."

"I am nowhere near that," I told him. "I eat healthy food every day, but just a lot less than I used to."

Back home, I kicked Scott's ass in Scrabble and he said no to a second round. Hah!

Upstairs in our bedroom a bit later, Peter laughed when I told him about the incident in the car. He hugged me so I couldn't get away and whispered, "Eat, my shrinking violet! Before I know it, you'll vanish!"

I thought that would be the end of Scott's interest in my food intake, but I'm wrong: for months, not a day goes by when he doesn't ask—often more than once—what I'm eating. He loves to cook and experiment with new recipes and gets so much pleasure from eating. Nothing wrong with that, especially since he's fit. I long for the same relationship with food, and I'm working toward that.

"Not eating is not the way to lose weight," he tells me again and again, almost with the same regularity as "How are you?"

I know he means well, but it's a source of constant bickering between us, which leads me to frequently lie to him about what I eat rather than defend it. Only six months ago, I would have used a friend's objection as a perfect excuse to quit the plan and resume a pigfest. *Oh, someone I like and trust doesn't approve of my diet? Screw this plan. Let's eat!*

But now nothing and no one will derail my determination. I adore Scott. I hope we will be friends forever, but he has never walked in my shoes. I am finally losing weight. I am proud of myself. *When you make the Shift, other people shift too—and sometimes they shift into nervous mode, criticizing mode, or sabotaging mode.* When it comes to doubters and naysayers, all you can do is stay the course.

16

I Can
(Eat Anything),
but I Don't

"One dessert won't kill you," says my accountant Dora at a restaurant near my office. She has just ordered strawberry shortcake and seems annoyed that I've passed on an after-dinner treat.

"You're probably right, but not today," I respond, a variation on what I have become used to saying when people tempt me to go out of bounds. It's almost as if subconsciously they are taunting the Fat Lady to see if they can get her to fail. Are Dora and others trying to sabotage my success? Are they jealous of my discipline? No way. I can't—and don't— believe they would do anything like that. Just as I find it hard to believe that anyone would tempt a recovering alcoholic by urging her to have a scotch.

But I know that it happens, especially when one person has an issue with drinking and doesn't want to own up to it. In some twisted way, it makes them feel better if they can get someone who is confronting their demons to slip. Looking back, that's *exactly* what I did with Peter when we were both on the Kirsch diet and he lost weight faster than I did. I was jealous of how quickly he was losing and I harangued him until ultimately I sabotaged his success. Dora's right: one dessert won't kill me, and I love her, but that attitude is what did me in all those years. Why tempt myself when I'm doing so well? Preference or priority.

My weight has been such a private, intimate issue for so long that it's an adjustment for me dealing with the unfamiliar scrutiny when it comes to what I'm eating or the change in my physical appearance. Friends and colleagues are one thing, but when it comes to strangers it feels a little creepy at first. As when the waitress at Seven's, a Turkish restaurant across from our office, all but rushes me, repeatedly, when our family walks in for dinner.

"So how much have you lost?" she asks loudly.

I usually just smile.

"Twenty? Thirty?" she persists.

"Maybe." I shrug.

Or when Joyce, the Chinese owner of the nail salon across the street, runs after Peter as he walks by. "How much Tory lose?"

On Facebook, where I post a couple thoughts daily, there's even less decorum and people are blunt: "Wow, you've lost a lot of weight. How much and how'd you do it?"

I would never think to ask that of anyone, no matter how curious I was, even if it was obvious that someone had shrunk to half her former size. But I learn to live with it and it's better than the withering look that people used to routinely give me, the one that all but shouted, "Wow, you've put on the feedbag, haven't you?" Or, God forbid, "Gaining or expecting?" These days, the comments about my weight take a very different tone.

A few weeks before, I joined *GMA*'s Robin Roberts and many other A-list women at the Eleventh Annual Women Who Care Luncheon benefiting United Cerebral Palsy. Robin is to receive an award from designer Diane Von Furstenberg, an ageless beauty. The lunch is at Cipriani on Forty-Second Street, a magnificent cathedral-domed venue across from Grand Central Station. At all these fancy social events, it's easy to avoid the food because everyone's talking, and our table is particularly obsessed with people watching, with women in every seat pointing out so and so. I stick to nibbling the grilled chicken on my plate, and when dessert is placed in front of me, instead of being the only one at the table to decline it, I simply ignore it. Robin turns to me and whispers, "I don't know what you're doing, but you look sensational." So unexpected, and coming from her, that compliment is infinitely sweeter than the decadent piece of chocolate staring up at me.

Now I'm steeling myself with Robin's words of encouragement as I await my *GMA* segment surrounded by tempting aromas from dishes that Emeril Lagasse has prepared. One of the perks of being at *GMA*'s Times Square studio at dawn is getting to meet a variety of A-list guests. I've always liked celebrity chefs who make frequent appearances—Emeril, Wolfgang Puck, Mario Batali—because they're funny and fun and, well, I love to eat.

However, post-Shift, I routinely resist the delicious cuts of grilled steaks, rich lasagna, or sinful desserts that are passed around on plates in the studio for all to taste. When Karen Pickus, *GMA*'s food stylist, offers me a scoop of Emeril's potato salad, my producer, Laura Zaccaro, who is well aware that I'm on the straight and narrow, looks to see how I'll handle it. I say no thanks. I tell her that I never eat before my segments, but she's no dummy. As she pulls back the plate, Karen whispers, "You're so good. You have to tell me your secret."

Well, Karen, the secret is pretty simple: I channel my inner Nancy Reagan and just say no. But I am often tempted to say yes—not because I am hungry for the food itself but to avoid the inevitable scrutiny, the "Oh, you're on a diet?" line of questioning. Sometimes, while it might be easier to acquiesce and please people around me, I have to remind myself that they are not going carry those extra pounds around. I am. So it comes right back again to pausing for a moment to reflect on preference or priority—and the stark line between them.

At the beginning, sacrifice is painful and at times agony. Just as the budding athlete, actor, or singer has moments when she

wants to quit, so too do I—a potential weight-loss champ—
have doubts in the middle of the day and night about whether
it's all worth it. But then I think about the alternative—
unraveling all that I've accomplished, reverting back to an
unhealthy life, being a lousy role model for my kids, losing
my *GMA* gig—and the sacrifice becomes all the more reasonable.

It helps when I think about the difference between two
words: "don't" and "can't." In the past, I followed rules that
were set by diet experts who dictated what I could or could
not eat. When I found myself at lunch or dinner with a friend
and she suggested something off-limits—let's say splitting a
plate of three-thousand-calorie butter, cheese, and bacon
spaghetti carbonara—I'd invariably blurt out, "Oh, no way.
I *can't* eat that."

I believed it in my heart and soul. But in the back of my
mind I resented it because no one likes to be *told* they *can't*
eat one food or another. I think it unleashed the rebel in me:
told to go right, I went left—simply out of spite.

"Sure you can," my friend would say, just as one kid might
try to convince another to do something that Mom had said
not to do under the strictest of orders. More often than not
when this happened, I'd give in and dig into that creamy
pasta or cheesecake. Don't tell *me* what I can't eat!

Adopting a "don't" as opposed to "can't" attitude empow-
ers me to make specific sacrifices. *With the Shift, I can eat
anything I want, but I* don't. I can resist cheating because I
just *don't* eat certain foods anymore. It's a choice that I have

made for *myself*, not one that someone has made *for me*. I can walk past a bakery, and instead of having a woe-is-me attitude—"Gee, I wish I *could* eat ten cupcakes, but my diet says I *can't*"—my mind-set is: "I *could* eat ten cupcakes but I *don't* eat them," because I am on a mission.

A few months after Emma and Jake were born, other moms would routinely ask how I managed two infants when all they could do was handle one. At first I didn't know how to respond, but I got used to saying, "Taking care of two babies is all I know. It's my reality." I think about those days when I ponder my current challenge. Early on I viewed myself as some sort of martyr who said no to anything tasty or fun—probably because I was still in a "can't" phase. Force of will and clarity around my goal played a huge role in resisting temptation. But now with some road behind me, making good choices isn't a sacrifice. It is for my benefit. This is my new normal—and it's much easier to manage with each passing moment. Taking care of myself is my reality.

The Big Three-O

t's just after 7 A.M. and I've slept later than I should have. But I wake up with great expectations: I have a hunch that I'm about to get some really good news. I kick off the covers and take the seven steps to the bathroom. My white Taylor scale is in its usual position. I pull my T-shirt over my head and wedge it into the towel rack. I stand on the scale, left foot first, which is the reverse of the right-foot-first superstition that Jake has made me promise to do when I board airplanes. *I've savored my victories in one-pound increments*, grateful as each bit of fat disappears from my body, but this could be a big one.

"Ahh!" I yell for Peter in a voice that's a cross between a squeal and a shriek as I open the door. I'm so excited that I almost forget to grab a towel to cover my naked body. Walking around in the buff is something that I never do, especially in broad daylight.

While my voice doesn't guarantee good news, the expression on my face is a dead giveaway as Peter approaches from down the hall.

"Lay it on me, sweetie." He smiles, having anticipated this moment he knows means so much to me.

"It's good. Really good."

"Hit me, mama."

I almost can't spit it out because it's the first time I've ever reached this kind of milestone.

"Thirty pounds. The big three-O!"

I want to cry as Peter gives me a tight hug that lasts longer than usual—as if pointedly trying to show me how much this moment resonates with him too. I still have so far to go, but I am proud that I've lost all this weight. In the shower, I start thinking about buying a piece of jewelry, a serious splurge on something expensive to mark my accomplishment. I wear the same stuff every day and don't look for new bling often, but losing thirty pounds is a first. The number seems huge and I want to reward myself.

But Peter has beat me to it, knowing for a while that my triple-ten moment was approaching. When I'm dressed and ready to go, he surprises me with a thin yellow gold bangle with bezel-set diamonds. I can tell this little sucker set him back. "Proud of you," he says, slipping it on my wrist. I'm impressed that he bought the bangle without any hints from

Emma, Mom, or me. I run my fingers around it and admire not only its simple beauty and the way it complements my other arm candy, but also how well it reflects the significance of my achievement. Just looking at it reinforces my determination to keep going.

"Thank you for standing by me for the last six months and helping me do what I never thought was possible," I tell him, holding his face in my hands. "You got me a bracelet, but you deserve a medal."

"Put that on the list," he says, kissing me.

I am pumped to do even more, eat even better, and finally get a good workout regimen going, even beyond my daily walks. It's one thing to lose some weight, but I know that if I am going to have a prayer of getting down to where I want to be and keeping it off, I'll have to move my ass more. Regularly. Also, I'm pushing forty-two, and I've read enough articles to know that heart disease kills many women, especially overweight and sedentary ones. Regular exercise can reverse that. I want to live a long, long time.

make the *Shift*

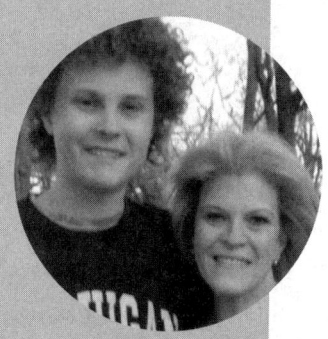

When I make the Shift, other people shift too—and sometimes they shift into nervous mode, criticizing mode, or sabotaging mode. I don't allow the naysayers and doubters to derail my determination.

With the Shift, I can eat anything I want, but I don't.

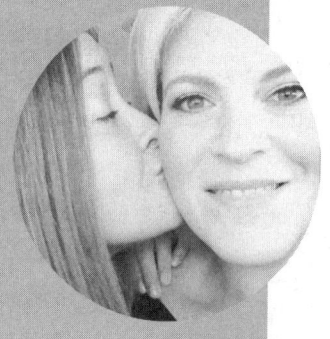

Savor your victories in one-pound increments.

MONTH 7

18

Shifts in My Marriage

With the Shift, I have sacrificed the foods I once craved the most. No one I know loves candy and chocolate more than I do, and yet I have gone for months without a single bite of either of them. Are there nights when I would love to dig into creamy, cheesy fettuccine Alfredo? Or a football-sized baked potato loaded with butter? Of course. But those choices are not in the stars for me now—and perhaps ever. And it's not just chocolate, pasta, and potatoes that I learn to do without.

On a dreary, rainy day like this one, I would love to go to a movie. Peter needs absolutely no excuse to go to one any day or night. He likes nothing more than sitting in a darkened theater in an aisle seat and zoning out. But on this Sunday morning, when he suggests we go see *Men in Black III*, I'm less than enthusiastic.

"What is with you and movies of late?" Peter asks. "I can't remember the last time we saw one together. Can you?"

I can't and I decide it's time to tell him the real reason I won't step into a theater today—or anytime soon. My determination is strong, but I also know my limits.

"Call me crazy, but I can't sit in a theater and not eat popcorn. And I'm definitely not going to torture myself listening to people chomp on something I can't have."

He stares at me and I'm not sure if he gets it or if he's going to lose it.

"I know you think I'm a whack job," I say. "But there it is."

Peter begins to suggest alternatives that he thinks will make the experience palatable. We'll find seats far away from everyone else. I can take a few pickles with me, maybe a couple of pieces of cheese and roasted almonds so my crunch is louder than theirs. He means well, but the thought of sitting for two hours while people gorge themselves on buckets of buttery popcorn and Buncha Crunch sounds awful. With each suggestion he makes, I shake my head no.

"Okay," Peter says, genuinely surprised that this is an issue. "Mind if I take Jake?"

In the coming months, the two boys see dozens of movies together while Emma and I do our thing. It works for everyone.

There are other shifts in my marriage too. We are in bed and Peter, who has slept in the buff every night since we've been together, is naked. I'm in my standard overnight attire: a V-neck T-shirt and black velour sweats. During last night's eleven o'clock news, Peter kissed me and I could tell that it would not have taken much effort on my part to go further. But I didn't and he didn't push it. Now the kids are still asleep and so is he, and we're cozy under a light summer comforter. Sliding out of my clothes, I press myself against his back, gently kissing his shoulder blades. I reach around his warm body to make small circles and figure eights with my fingers on his chest and stomach. He's always had the softest silky-smooth skin that rivals a baby's. As he stirs, I let my hand drift down. Soon my mouth goes there too, and before long I'm on top of him. As the sun rises, we are the happiest people on West Eighty-Sixth Street.

We have a lot of sex these days, but it's different than it used to be. Peter has always had a very healthy sex drive, probably the only area where my appetite fell short of his. Our record of intimacy is robust: I want to please him and he gladly returns the favor. But for years—the entirety of our eighteen-year marriage—I felt vulnerable, embarrassed, and anxious about being naked with my own husband. Disgust with my weight often stopped me from making overtures to him. He sensed it and didn't initiate sex every time he wanted to. I know this because we've discussed it since I made the Shift and have dropped in size. Just as I undressed in the bathroom with the door closed, so too did I insist that the lights be out and the room dark during sex, fearing Peter's interest in me would fizzle if he really knew what my naked body looked like.

Forget that he knew exactly what it looked like since a room only gets so dark. And lying naked with me over the course of nearly two decades—even in a pitch black room—gave him a very accurate picture. Never mind that Peter told me routinely that he didn't care whether I was fat or thin, that I was unnecessarily torturing myself by worrying about it and putting so much effort into hiding my body. He loved making love to me, and he reassured me whenever the subject came up: "Let me show you, right now," he'd say. Much of that fell on deaf ears. I felt so awkward and unattractive; I just couldn't believe that he could find me appealing.

All of that changed about a month ago. Peter and I had been separated for a week while he drove from Seattle to Chicago, where I was meeting him, in a Chevy Suburban SUV wrapped with a larger-than-life-sized image of me along with colorful graphics promoting our Spark & Hustle tour. He had been hauling all the staging for each of the conferences throughout the country and enjoying seeing parts of America that he'd never visited, while I flew back to New York between events to see the kids and appear on *GMA*. My flight to O'Hare landed early, and I had three hours to kill before Peter arrived.

We were staying at the James, a boutique hotel right off the Magnificent Mile, so I decided to take a stroll and window-shop. Walking along Michigan Avenue, I stopped in Victoria's Secret to browse for bras and undies, but I wound up walking out with a barely there lace nightie—the kind of number that probably wouldn't be worn all night if things went as planned. But this wasn't night. It was 1 P.M. when I greeted Peter with the shades drawn in our room and a black-fig-and-honey-scented Nest travel candle burning on the desk across from the bed where I was waiting.

"Whoa, baby," he said, as he left his bag by the door, kicked off his sneaks, and unbuttoned his shorts, which dropped to the floor. "To what do I owe this surprise?"

"Call it my fab forty moment," I said. "Close to forty pounds gone and I'm ready for some good lovin'."

Incredibly and unbelievably, all of my fear and modesty has vanished. *With every pound I've lost comes a corresponding increase in confidence about my body,* which translates into no longer having any problem dressing or undressing in front of Peter. Now during sex, instead of worrying about my most vulnerable body part, my stomach, and putting my hands over it in shame, I let him look. So far he hasn't run away.

Don't get me wrong, I still have miles to go in terms of completely embracing my body, and I trust that day will come. But when I look in the mirror, I'm happy to see a neck and a waistline that have definition—even if I am hardly ready to put on a pair of Daisy Dukes and walk down any street. And there's no way I'd wear a tank top in public now. A bathing suit in front of strangers? Not a chance. My thighs and arms still need tons of work. But for me, being able to foresee the day when I have a truly positive body image is a major victory, because for so many years that thought was so out there, so fantastic—as in a fantasy. A revved-up sex life is an unexpected dividend for losing a lot of weight.

I think of myself on our wedding day, happy but dressed in a navy suit, convinced that even on this day, which was just about Peter and me, decorum required me to present to the world the most covered-up version of myself. Sometimes I wish I could go back in time and talk to my twenty-three-year-old self, tell her to go ahead and wear the white dress. I want to tell her that the man she is marrying loves her with a passion that will not wane. I want to congratulate her on choosing a good husband, and I want to tell her she has as much control over choosing what she eats and how often she exercises. I wish I could give my twenty-three-year-old self the gift of the Shift. I would urge her to do *whatever it takes* to make herself feel and look better. To let her know that her dress size is not her destiny and that things *will* change, even if it seems to take forever. But all I can do is thank her. She did the best with what she had—mentally, emotionally, physically. She chose the husband who has been her partner and best friend. As Peter and I slip from the whispers of intimacy to talking about the everyday logistics that is the stuff of married life, I know the part of me that loves him most is that young girl who didn't know how to lose weight but knew how to recognize real love when she saw it.

make the *Shift*

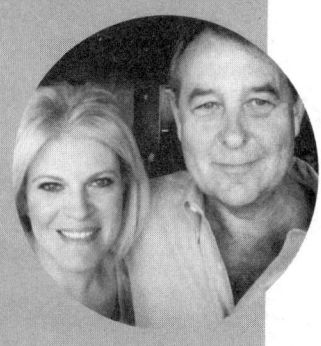

With every pound lost comes a corresponding increase in confidence.

MONTH 8

19

Ain't No Mountain
High Enough

W e never intended to buy a country house. But by chance Peter met a woman named Judy who was walking her Lab near our apartment. "Nice dog," he said, and they became fast friends. About a year later she told him that her house in the Catskills had become too much for her to handle and she was selling it.

"Big place?" Peter asked, assuming it was.

"No, just a little cottage," Judy said.

Intrigued, especially when she told him the two-bedroom place overlooked an apple orchard, had a thirty-mile view of the valley, and sat on a private lake, Peter arranged for us to see it that weekend. On the seventy-two-mile drive, I thought Peter had lost his mind.

"Why are we doing this?" I asked.

"Hey, if it's a dump at least we had a day in the country," he replied.

As we turned onto Altamont Road in Bloomingburg, there was a small, pristine white house surrounded by beautiful maple trees. Judy was playing with Oliver on the front lawn, and an elderly man was sitting on the screened-in porch.

"We're buying this," we both said in unison, and we did about a month later. Not only did we fall in love with the rustic house that weekend, but Peter got a bonus. Judy introduced us to her friend who was visiting: actor Abe Vigoda, who played Tessio in *The Godfather* (Peter's favorite movie) and Fish on TV's *Barney Miller*. In the past sixteen years we've renovated the kitchen; added bathrooms and bedrooms; and knocked down walls to make an open living space where everyone hangs out. It's our little piece of heaven away from the hectic city.

On this August day, I find myself in unfamiliar territory, facing Peter across the threadbare and drooping net on one of the two tennis courts at the town park down the hill from our house. The courts have seen better days: the green surface has cracked in many places, allowing weeds to sprout. I'm only here because nobody else is and because of some arm-twisting by Peter, who has brought a large plastic bucket filled with a few dozen yellow tennis balls. A good thing too, since many of them end up sailing over the fence and attracting burrs in the tall grass. But to Peter's (and my) amazement, I manage plenty of decent volleys.

"Hey, you know you're not bad," he says, genuinely impressed that I can hit a tennis ball across the net, let alone return a shot—a skill I learned in summer camp as a kid. We find ourselves back here a handful of times throughout the summer, alternately laughing and taking our competition seriously—I more than Peter. It's a good thing we don't keep score: he really knows how to play.

A few years earlier we had put in a sleek pool at the house, our smartest investment, but I've never done anything more than spend hours floating in it. Now I make a point of moving around. I do laps and tread water in the deep end while Peter and I talk. Nothing that would impress Michael Phelps, of course, but for me it's a lot more than taking a bath in an oversized tub.

"Hey, you want to walk to the hardware store? I need a few things," Peter says to me as I'm poolside the next morning reading *People* magazine.

"That's, like, three miles away," I say, none too interested.

"Six, if we walk there and back," Peter says. "Be something to do. We never walk anywhere around here."

It's true. We drive pretty much everywhere, even to the lake, which is a four-minute walk . . . downhill. It's never occurred to us to walk anywhere. But an hour later we've reached the bottom of the mountain and are heading along Winterton Road toward the village. We've taken back roads, and even though it's mostly downhill, there are many steep parts and even some uphill portions. I notice houses and barns and details that I have driven past hundreds of times but ignored until now. With each turn, seeing my face flush in the summer heat, Peter says we are almost there. But the distance—or at least the time it would take us to walk it—is longer than either of us anticipated. It's almost noon, the sun is blazing, and neither of us thought to bring water.

"*Something to do!*" I pant at Peter, who says, "Just a bit farther."

I didn't wear socks—I never do—and I feel blisters forming. Peter immediately takes off his and hands them to me to put on.

I'm going to keel over. This is a disaster. Why don't *any* of these passing drivers realize that I'm about to collapse and offer us a ride before I have a heat stroke?

Finally, shortly after noon, we get to the hardware store and Peter buys a couple things while I pour myself on the bench out front where the bus to New York stops a few times a day. I sit there staring at nothing, numb. He returns with two bottles of cold water.

"There's no way I can climb back up that mountain," I tell him. It's too hot and I am beat. My shirt is drenched with sweat and my hair is a damp, frizzy mess from the humidity. Some women were made for this. I am not one of them.

"No problem," Peter says, pointing to our Honda parked nearby. David, visiting for the weekend with his wife, Julie, and baby Charlotte, cooked up this charade with Peter at breakfast. They drove down earlier and dropped off our car so it would be waiting for us. Peter knew damn well I could walk down the mountain but not back again.

"Hey, how about Twin Cone?" Peter asks as I position the car's air-conditioning vents to blow in my face.

"And reverse whatever good this forced march accomplished?" I respond, exasperated by his good humor, the mere suggestion of getting ice cream, this unbelievably painful trek, and, well, everything. "We are never doing this again."

Yet somehow on subsequent weekends when David and Julie visit, Peter convinces me to walk down the mountain again, then calls David to pick us up at the bottom. One time, to shake it up, Julie—after privately asking if I'm really okay with it because she always has my back—drives us down and we walk back up Mountain Road—at a thirty-degree incline. "Never again," I say when we finally get home and I fall in the pool and sit motionless for hours. But eventually, after a few rough outings, I come to look forward to our weekend treks, and we find other roads and well-traveled trails in the woods to check out. It's a chance for us to talk without interruption—I leave my iPhone at home, a rarity—and we become walking real estate speculators by evaluating each house we pass: "tear down, "remodel," or "gut."

Who knew I could become a hiker? Not me, that's for sure. *Suddenly anything seems possible.* I discover a joy in the country that I hadn't experienced before. For as long as we've owned it, I've viewed this as a place to zone out, unwind, and do a whole lot of nothing. Now it becomes a healthy haven where I explore nature and push myself through the great outdoors.

20

Today, I Am a Medium

Back in the city a week later, I am walking by the Alvin Ailey American Dance Theater on West Fifty-Fifth Street, and I see a dozen or so women taking a class and I think, *What if?* If I can hike and play tennis, is it possible that I could be a *dancer?* Not everyone is pencil thin, yet they appear to be so beautiful and graceful in their tights. *I want to be just like them, to focus on doing my best as opposed to obsessing over what I'd look like in that stretchy outfit,* dancing clumsily, as women around me move so effortlessly. I haven't joined a gym or taken an exercise class because I still don't want to be the slow girl in the back who sticks out like a sore thumb. Someday I think I could participate in a class and not feel totally self-conscious, but I'm not there yet.

Back in the office with dancer daydreams still flitting around my head, Gianna is waiting for me. She helps coordinate my television segments and tells me that a company wants to send a sample jacket for me to consider wearing on-air. "They come in extra small through double XL."

"Well, I definitely don't need a double XL anymore, thank God," I say. "But ask them to send an XL to be safe."

That's when Dora, our accountant, turns to me with a puzzled look: "You still think you're huge, don't you? I mean, not that you were ever huge . . ." She gets momentarily tongue-tied but then resumes. "You're definitely not an extra large. You're not even a large. If I had to bet, I'd say you could wear a medium in whatever jacket it is."

Realizing it's a sensitive subject, Gianna jumps in and says she'll get a range of sizes, and three hours later a messenger arrives for my moment of truth. I grab the XL first—I'm swimming in it.

"See," Dora says, now confident. "Skip the large and just go to what I said in the first place." So I do as she suggests and the medium fits perfectly. Without skipping a beat, Dora says, "You have a distorted image of your body."

"Come again?" I say, not quite sure what she is getting at.

"When I lose weight, I continue to think I'm bigger than I am," Dora says. "I've noticed the same thing with you. You cling to what *was*, not what *is*. You still think you're fat, but you're not."

I begin to realize that I *could* be in that Alvin Ailey class, that my image is worse than my reality, and that I've got to get back to being the optimist I've always been. In business I know that negativity gets me nowhere and that I thrive on positive thinking. I have to do better at applying that logic to myself too.

This is reinforced when I'm in the dressing room at Banana Republic and about to try on a pair of size 10 black cotton cropped pants even though I know full-length pants are more flattering because they elongate my legs and, at just five feet four inches, I can use the lift. Like the XL jacket I tried on in the office just days earlier, these pants are huge. I'm stunned. It must be the style.

"Need any help?" the salesgirl asks through the door.

"Yeah, actually, would you please bring me an eight?" I'm practically whispering since I've always refused help of any kind, ashamed of my size and not eager to share it with anyone. Who wants to tell the skinny salesgirl—they're all skinny—to bring around a bigger size? Or worse, try on the largest size and find that I can't quite close the zipper. Just the humiliating memory of those occasions—many—gives me goose bumps.

Now I'm blown away that I'm about to slip into an 8. To my amazement, even the 8 is loose. *No way,* I say to myself. I'm about to buy them, figuring they'll shrink when washed, but then I decide to go for gold. In a laughable move prompted by what must be some kind of subconscious desire to punish myself, I ask the salesgirl to get me a 6.

"There's no chance they'll fit, but I want to see the difference," I tell her. How many times has she heard *that* pathetic line? When I try on the pants, tears stream down my face as I stand in front of the three-way mirror. Never in my adult life have I come *close* to wearing a size 6. I know Banana Republic runs generously—it's hardly a couture cut—but a 6 is a 6! I want to start spreading the news. Post this on Facebook. I'm ready to tweet. This moment is Instagram worthy. The store should make an announcement on its public address system: *The Fat Girl fits into a 6!*

I pay for the pants, grinning uncontrollably as I swipe my AmEx card at the register with extra gusto, oblivious to anyone or anything. As I walk out into the hot sun that is baking Broadway, I have flashbacks of walking several blocks all those days when I really would have preferred to take a taxi. Then, as if some higher power is high-fiving me, I pass a faded quote from supermodel Kate Moss posted in the window of a tacky P90X studio. I never imagined words like these would ever resonate with me: "Nothing tastes as good as skinny feels."

The next week I get another encouraging email from Barbara. "You look fantastic. Coffee or lunch soon?"

In January, no one could have ever convinced me that by summer, I'd be receiving complimentary notes from the head of talent at ABC News, climbing up and down (okay, mostly down) mountain roads, and fitting into normal clothing that's always been off limits.

Shift Happens

21

Our family has split up.

Emma and I are seated next to each other on an American Airlines flight to Los Angeles. Last we heard, Peter and Jake had stopped for lunch at a diner in Rhode Island on their way to Cape Cod for some fishing and golf. The kids thought this up. Between sleepaway camp for a month and putting up with my busy travel schedule, Emma felt we all missed out on time together. Also, having turned fifteen a few months ago, she thought it'd be a blast if she and Jake each got a fantasy trip to cap the summer—I would take Emma wherever she wanted, within reason, and Peter would take Jake to his chosen destination. True to their personalities, we're on opposite coasts.

I have used frequent flier miles to upgrade to business class, where my celebrity-obsessed daughter prays we'll be seated near a Kardashian or Jenner. Instead, a few older men are reading newspapers, working on their laptops, or sleeping. For this four-day trip Emma has asked—begged, actually— that I suspend all diet talk and just indulge.

"Of course," I say without thinking. I feel guilty. I've been on the road for work even more than usual this summer, away from home a lot, and I promised to give her whatever she wants on this trip. But I tell her that celebrities don't in- dulge as much foodwise as she thinks. "Does Britney Spears get her hot bod eating at Sonic every day? Think she doesn't spend endless hours working out?"

Emma brushes me off. "I thought you said you were good with my whole fantasy thing."

"I'm good, baby," I say, slicing a bit of filet mignon that we've both chosen for lunch. For dessert she has an ice-cream sundae with hot chocolate, nuts, and strawberries. I pass, but eye it lustfully.

On the bumper-to-bumper ride along the 405 to Beverly Hills, Emma blares Z100. She talks nonstop about how ex- cited she is and what fun we're going to have, going over the list for the umpteenth time of exactly what we're going to do every waking moment. I'm getting more and more caught up in her giddiness and the escape this weekend promises.

We turn off Sunset Boulevard and pull into the driveway of the storied hundred-year-old pink Beverly Hills Hotel— home to the stars and site of the iconic Polo Lounge, named after polo-playing guests of the 1940s. We feel like celebrities ourselves at the hotel as we walk past the famous bungalows through a landscape of lush, tropical plants.

Our room is large, with a sitting area, giant TV, walk-in closet, and bathroom featuring double sinks and a tub big enough for Emma and me to soak in. I can't help but notice a scale. I instantly decide I'll ignore it, the first time in eight months when I won't be weighing myself first thing in the morning. It looks old and a tad rickety anyway, I tell myself, which means it's probably unreliable. Or maybe I'm just talking myself into thinking that. Maybe I need a break from the scale—a break in general. God knows I have been a very good girl for what seems like an eternity. I am so proud of my discipline and results. It wouldn't kill me to loosen the reins a little bit. I tell myself I'm going to accede to Emma's every wish, but I'm not going lose *all* control: after all, I *am* the grown-up here.

We walk around the grounds and check out the pool— quiet, with only a few people sunbathing—then head to the Ivy on North Robertson Boulevard, named for its ivy-covered exterior walls. A top celebrity hangout, it draws hundreds of A-listers each week. Dozens of paparazzi loiter full time in front to shoot photos as they exit their Mercedeses, Hummers, and BMWs. This is the bistro where John Travolta and Danny DeVito had a funny lunch in *Get Shorty*. In *The Bodyguard*, Kevin Costner and Whitney Houston are exiting from the Ivy when a little girl and her mom ask for an autograph. Scenes from HBO's *Entourage* have been shot here with the boys having a casual meal. But on this day all the stars we'd recognize are nowhere to be found. Oh well.

Emma and I each have a chopped salad and split the Ivy's famous onion rings, battered lightly and deep-fried to crispy perfection. Sinful. I haven't tasted a fried anything or poured ketchup—pure sugar dressed in tomato flavoring—on anything for so long. Oh, how I've missed that Heinz. For a second as we leave the restaurant, I regret eating those heavenly rings, but then I think: *If I'm going to be bad, let it be on the first day. Tomorrow I'll do better.*

We spend the rest of the day shopping, popping into boutiques along Robertson and nearby streets. I'm tempted to suggest we go back to the hotel and call it a night—it's almost midnight East Coast time—but the sun is barely setting and there's little chance Emma wants to head back anytime soon. She has energy to burn, and after all those onion rings, the last thing I should do is lie down and sleep. Better to keep moving.

Seeing as we had a late lunch, I suggest we skip dinner and just go straight for dessert. I'm thinking I'm being prudent: if we have dinner, Emma will demand dessert anyway, which would make this day a true caloric disaster. She's fine with just dessert, a typical teenager. So we head to Millions of Milkshakes on Santa Monica Boulevard, which is on Emma's must-visit list because she has read that stars hit this design-your-own-shake hot spot often. But all we find is a guy behind the counter who welcomes us with a loud, "Hey, girls," and grabs an empty blender.

"Nutella. Cookie dough. Reese's Peanut Butter Cups. Kit Kat," I say by rote, as if nothing about my eating habits has changed whatsoever. I haven't had a speck of chocolate—*nada*—in more than seven months, and the specter of what I'm about to taste gives me a terrific rush. The one you get when you know you're about to do something you really shouldn't do but you just can't help yourself—mainly because you don't want to. The idea of bending the rules and giving in to temptation makes me feel positively, dangerously wild.

"Whipped cream?"

I nod, as if to say, *Duh!*

We read somewhere online that the typical Millions drink has eleven hundred calories, but the shake we share is no doubt double that—and we slurp down every last drop. On the ride back to the hotel I get quiet, and Emma asks me if anything is wrong.

"Not at all, baby," I lie. "Just thinking about work for a second." What I'm really thinking is what an idiot I was: we could have had a healthy dinner, and even if Emma wanted dessert, I could have passed on it. Just because a kid says we're not going to think at all about what we eat does not mean her mother must follow blindly. And yet I do anyway, feeling unnervingly free to let loose a little bit after being good for so long.

Peter calls and says he and Jake spent the day fishing off Harwich and both of them caught lots of large striped bass. They've just returned from dinner at Rookies, a pizza place that Peter has been going to since he was a kid.

"As good as always," Peter says. "Speaking of food, how you doing?" he asks without needing to elaborate.

"Don't ask," I say, and we both laugh. I'm too exhausted to beat myself up.

A few minutes later Jake texts photos of him holding fish that are half as big as he is. "Check this out, Mom. Playing golf tomorrow. Love you." Sounds like all's well with my boys.

The next day I drive around showing Emma some of the sights. We head north on the Pacific Coast Highway to Malibu and check out all the pricey beach houses overlooking the ocean. From there we drive back to Hollywood, where we take a photo of ourselves with the iconic HOLLYWOOD sign behind us. I ask if she wants to stroll along the fifteen blocks of the Hollywood Walk of Fame, but once she spots the Spanish-style Roosevelt Hotel—a famous Hollywood haunt—we decide to have lunch there. Emma feels like a hamburger with fries and so do I, but remembering my brief chat with Peter last night, I order mine without a bun and a side salad instead of fries. I've gotten very good at speaking up to waiters to ask them to remove bread from the table, hold things like croutons on salads, and change my order if necessary. Most are very accommodating. I remember one dinner where I was looking forward to having the creamed spinach until I ask about the specific ingredients and the waiter told me it included flour. This time when the waitress leaves, after I've nixed the bun and fries, Emma shoots me a look that shouts, *Lighten up!*, to which I give her a silent not-to-worry signal. When Emma's plate arrives—looking a lot more inviting than my plain patty with some greens next to it—I pick at her fries. So much for being good.

In the early evening, we head back to our room to change, then go down to the Polo Lounge to meet my friend Melissa for drinks—water for me, Shirley Temple for Emma. I think the crowded bar has good vibes until I see a woman who is smiling nervously at me—just short of a stare. This goes on for a few minutes until she comes over and says she knows me from *GMA* and likes my segments.

"If you're the only person here who anyone recognizes, we're in big trouble, Mom," Emma says, and she's not kidding. My daughter has come here to see stars, not women who recognize me.

Afterward it's dinner at Wolfgang Puck's Steakhouse in the lobby of the Beverly Wilshire Hotel, the setting of one of my favorite movies, *Pretty Woman*. Since I've featured Puck's kitchen and cooking products many times on *GMA*, I called his rep to ask which of Wolfgang's spots he'd recommend. This was the place, and he made the reservation. I think that's the extent of his courtesy, but he arranges the royal treatment, which is apparent the second I give the maître d' my name.

Our waiter encourages us to sample anything and everything. "On the house," he says with a bright smile. I appreciate the gesture but instead of going crazy we order a tuna tartare appetizer, then share a filet with sides of truffle mushrooms and spinach. But when the bread basket comes around every fifteen minutes, piled high with new offerings, we can't help ourselves. Actually, we *do* help ourselves. That buttery pretzel bread: Oh . . . my . . . god.

Ten minutes after we're seated in a prime people-watching spot, actor Danny DeVito arrives and takes a booth near us. Emma definitely recognizes him and hopes this is a sign of things to come. But she is not impressed to see an actor who could easily be her grandfather. "He doesn't count, Mom. I want stars *under* sixty." My baby ain't easy to please.

When we get back to our room, I receive a text from Scott in New York saying that he's seen our pictures on Facebook and it looks like we're having a blast.

"But are you EATING in La-La Land?" he asks.

"More than you can imagine," I write back.

"Great," responds Scott, my diet guardian angel.

Now with Emma sleeping beside me in our king bed, I feel stuffed after an elaborate dinner—an unfamiliar feeling after months of carefully watching what I eat. For a moment I panic when I think about how much I have crossed the line.

"Go to sleep, Mom," Emma whispers, and I turn off the TV and drift off.

On Day Three, after some fun shopping, I suggest we grab salads for lunch.

"Gotta go to In-N-Out Burger while we're here. YOLO, Mom," Emma says, using the teen shorthand for You Only Live Once, and we're off.

"I love you, Mommy," Emma says for no reason a few minutes later, momentarily stopping her lip sync to a One Direction tune as she copilots from her charcoal leather seat, eyeing me from behind her Ray-Ban aviator sunglasses. She is having a great time. I'm happy.

At In-N-Out I employ the classic diet trick of ordering lettuce-wrapped burgers, which aren't on the menu but they'll make them if you ask. Emma likes that idea, but of course we compensate for not having buns by ordering animal fries loaded with mayo, Thousand Island dressing, cheese, and grilled onions. Just a few thousand extra calories.

Midafternoon we stop at Sprinkles Cupcakes, a bakery on Santa Monica Boulevard. I love the business, having met owner Candace Nelson at *GMA* just a few weeks earlier where I found her so likable and smart. Emma orders red velvet ice cream between a sliced red velvet cupcake. I go for chocolate espresso ice cream, my first scoop all year. Scott would be so proud of me right now.

We are obsessed with Sprinkles' outdoor vending machine that lets you purchase a cupcake at any hour of the day and tell each other we'll be back for a midnight snack. We wind up never doing it—partially because I know that would cross into binging. I'm walking a thin line here: worried about how much I'm eating but not wanting Emma to explode if I suggest watching our food intake. I'm by no means eating as much as I did pre-Shift but a lot more than I normally would these days. God help me if I broach restraint anytime soon.

. . .

On our last full day, we have lunch at Joan's on Third, where we start with chicken, Brie, and grilled onions on focaccia bread—melted to perfection with cheese oozing from the sides—then sample an assortment of pasta salads and butternut squash. For dessert we have cappuccinos and split a chocolate coffee cake. We're so full, but within a few hours Emma is somehow hungry again, plus we have another hot spot on her list to visit. I think about suggesting something else—*How about we go back to see those stars on the Hollywood Walk of Fame?*—but before I can open my mouth Emma says we're going to Lemonade. The hot spot on Beverly Boulevard is part lemonade stand, part grade-school cafeteria. The place is packed with moms and daughters like us, but Emma is a little bummed that none of them are *famous* moms and daughters. Every single person in line is thin. I can't find anyone who's overweight—not even behind the counter. Maybe this stuff isn't so bad after all. Or am I trying to justify another splurge?

We order strawberry lemonade and a selection of sides: Brussels sprouts with shaved ricotta, an amazing roasted cauliflower dish, purple cabbage, and a slice of red velvet cake with cream cheese frosting, which Emma enjoys but I don't touch. Not that I've suddenly found religion, I'm just not into red velvet. But in the back of my mind I'm happy Emma picked the red velvet cake so I can avoid temptation, because I have gone overboard these past few days. Seriously, utterly, and completely overboard. And I know there will be a price to pay for it. Soon.

I wish I had brought my Nike FuelBand, a bracelet that tracks how many steps I take and calories I burn. I have come to rely on it because it reminds me in clear digital numbers when I've spent the whole day sitting at my desk and when I've been up and about. A day when I take two thousand steps is a bad, sedentary one; anything over ten thousand is good because it means I'm moving. Not much I can do about it now.

Our last dinner is Japanese—a relatively safe choice with edamame, house salads, and tuna sashimi. Emma spends the entire meal rubbernecking. Sadly there is no star in sight. How is it that we've struck out everywhere—with the exception of DeVito, who she says doesn't count? We head back to the hotel and pack for our early flight home the next morning. I'm glad to be tired, since sleep will prevent me from obsessing on what's to come: my reunion with the scale. I doze off, content that Emma has had a blast but worried about weight repercussions clouding the trip. I have been a bad girl.

On the drive to LAX, Emma and I are both talking about how we had *the best time*, a major mother-daughter bonding experience that we'll remember forever. In so many ways, the famous hotel and all the shopping and trendy eateries *were* a total fantasy, especially for an East Coast teenager obsessed with all things LA chic. The last photo we take is of us smiling at the iconic Beverly Hills sign made famous in *The Beverly Hillbillies*.

On the plane, I tell Emma, "The celeb sighting was a bust, but otherwise you had a good time, right, sweetie?"

"I had an amazing time and really appreciate you doing this for me. You're the best mom ever," she says, reaching over to kiss me on the cheek as the plane taxis to the runway. I can tell she means it and my heart swells. These are the moments moms live for. Once we're in the air, she reclines her seat for a nap. I watch her sleep, overcome with love for my little girl.

As Emma snoozes, I begin to think about all the work I have ignored and things on my plate next week. But it's all quickly overshadowed when I realize what I've just done. No, I didn't go completely crazy and gorge myself mindlessly like I normally would have on a pre-Shift vacation. This was definitely more reserved, but nonetheless I have veered way off course, a diet detour equivalent to flying from New York to Miami via Minneapolis, or perhaps British Columbia. Sure, we shared many plates, but I also went deep into the Danger Zone and reintroduced all kinds of carbs, fat, and junk into my body—things I had successfully avoided for months. My disappointment in myself puts me in a funk.

But then it occurs to me that Emma and I did a fair amount of walking and we weren't sitting nearly as much as I normally do in the office. Maybe I'll be okay.

Being away from home was no excuse for cheating because I had just recently proved that I could do it. So far this year, I had logged forty-one thousand frequent flier miles traveling back and forth to eighteen cities for my Spark & Hustle events. I was stuck in airports where fast-food chains rule and traveled on interstate highways where food choices were no better. I ate out for every single meal and could have gotten myself into a bunch of trouble. Nobody would have blamed me.

But I managed to still lose weight on the road through a combination of making good food choices, avoiding bad ones, and moving more than I would have sitting behind my desk. When forced to stop at a greasy joint, I chose a burger patty without the bread. I often used Yelp and Urbanspoon to help us find local restaurants off the beaten path with healthier options. And we purposely served chicken salads for lunch at our events because I knew they worked for me— and my staff agreed that everyone likes them. I was so busy running the events that it wasn't difficult staying away from all the candy we set out on tables. Ditto for the warm oatmeal and chocolate chip cookies we served every afternoon.

It's a reminder of the truism that has helped me so much over the past eight months: *preference or priority.* It is my priority to stay true to my Shift, but this time it was my preference to enjoy a girls' getaway trip with my daughter, calories be damned. I can only hope that this one swing backward won't completely derail my hard work so far.

22

Getting Back in the Groove

want badly to get back in the groove. As Emma sleeps beside me, I pull out a journal that I kept during my recent Spark & Hustle tour. I start flipping through and reminiscing about all the inspiring women I met who graced our stage. Here's an entry from May 22 in New York, where Carol's Daughter founder Lisa Price talked about how introspection—looking at what you're doing right and wrong—is good for the soul. I wrote: *She had one of the most powerful moments of the day, telling 500 women in our audience, "When problems crop up, be comfortable turning the mirror on yourself." It's so empowering to know that **each of us has the power to fix whatever's gone wrong.*** Amen to that, I think, because I am determined to right all the wrongs from this food fest of mine.

At that same event, Barbara Bradley Baekgaard, cofounder of Vera Bradley, talked about the power of nice. "We don't hire nice people and tell them to be nice. We only hire nice people." I realize that my Shift has made me nicer because I'm happier and more content with myself these days. There continue to be so many moments to privately celebrate my good choices, which keep me smiling.

I flip to an entry from a week later in Los Angeles where I reflect on self-esteem expert Jess Weiner's definition of fear—"It's a down payment on a debt you may not owe." I wrote: *My takeaway is* **to listen to the fear, but refuse to allow it to paralyze me.** So many times in my life I have let fear— particularly the fear of failing at a diet—immobilize me. I'd fall off the wagon and quickly lose all hope. Not this time.

Anastasia Soare's story of how she became the eyebrow guru makes all my struggles pale in comparison. I wrote: *She came to this country from Romania about twenty years ago, not speaking English and without a support system. She joked that she didn't even know how to sign a check. Now she has brow studios everywhere you turn. She's truly living the American dream, which she says anyone can do. "Be prepared to work hard." That's how she summed it up. God knows I get that concept.* The next month in Washington, D.C., the founders of Georgetown Cupcake impressed me with their warning that if you wait for the perfect time to take action, you may be waiting forever: *Once Katherine and Sophie realized this, they* **embraced the beauty of the chaos.** *I have to do more of that,* my entry said.

On June 7 in Minneapolis, I was blown away by firecracker

Rhoda Olsen, CEO of Great Clips, a hair salon chain. I wrote: *She was more fit than most people in the room. She attributed her extraordinary business success in large part to her physical stamina. She works out daily and holds push-up contests in the office. It's even more remarkable given that she's turning 60.* If that's not motivation to move my butt even more, I'm not sure what is.

And if anyone was able to sum up what I have felt so many times in the past eight months, it was Gigi Butler, who on June 27 in Nashville told us how she had a baby, raised her alone, and expanded her cupcake franchise to more than sixty locations in nineteen states, racking up $30 million in sales. *When one woman stood up to ask how exactly she manages to make it all happen without losing her mind, Gigi paused. I couldn't tell if she was pissed at the question. But then she said,* **"You just have to suck it up."** *That is totally my new mantra now. Oh, how I love that.*

I'm not whining about doing without my favorite foods. I'm dealing with it just fine because that's the only option. But I also liked the message from Pam Turkin, owner of Just Baked, a cupcake chain, on July 26 in Detroit. *She said, "A business plan is only as good as the day it's written." So true. And the same could be said for this whole Shift of mine. The plan is worthless if I don't stick to it. Now even more thrilled I didn't touch the 12 cupcakes she gave me.*

And finally, just a few weeks ago in Phoenix, health and wellness expert Chris Freytag prompted me to take a long walk at sunset. *She said,* **"Make time for what's most**

***important to you. There's always someone busier than you
and they manage to get it done."*** *Hearing that inspired me to
put on my sneakers and get outside for an hour at the end of the
event since I had time to kill before my flight. Normally I would
have napped or played on Facebook. Of course I would have said
there was no time to exercise. I'm going to post her words on my
desk.*

Reading my journal calms me down a bit, but when Peter
calls as soon as we are back and suggests we all go out to dinner to celebrate being together again, I cut him off. "Not a
chance, no way." Before he can ask why, I say I'm on the
other line with my mom and can't talk.

Mom is not on the other line, but right before Peter's call I
was thinking it was time to face the music: my little white
scale is in the same place I left it, under the sink in my bathroom. I pull it out, left foot first, then right.

Argh.

On this West Coast fantasy trip, I have gained six pounds
in the span of just ninety-six hours, wrecking what had taken
me more than a month to accomplish. Not that I need more
bad news, but when I sit down to pee I know just how much I
have screwed up. One thing that's kept me on track are Ketostix, small plastic strips available in drugstores that mea-
sure ketones in urine. I discovered them during my Atkins
phase when I read that ketones are produced as your body
burns fat for fuel, which is exactly what happens when few
or no carbs are present. Better to burn fat than to store it.
Since January I haven't missed a day of peeing on the teeny

padded edge of a strip, the spot that's chemically designed to detect ketones. Fifteen seconds later I check the color: purple is the jackpot because it means my system is burning fat since there's hardly a carb in sight. But if the small square is faded beige, I've exceeded my carb limit and I must get myself back on track. Even when I know I'm toeing the line perfectly, I never tire of the thrill of seeing that eggplant color quickly appear. I'm obsessive about my Ketostix routine because the strips help keep me honest.

Even though a six-pound gain is a sure bet that my strip will be off-white, I want to see it myself. The result is devastating, so light in color that there's not even a trace of pale pink. The worst. I have no regrets about spending uninterrupted time with Emma, but I'm kicking myself for not bringing these strips with me on the trip. They would have stopped me from letting things get so out of control. How could I have abandoned something that kept me straight for so long?

Emma's already on her iPhone, talking excitedly to her friends about the trip, as I sit in my bedroom and freak out about the enormity of what has transpired. This is one big Shift storm and it's all my fault. I think about calling Peter back and saying that dinner out might actually be a good idea. Then just as quickly, I think, *No way.* I am not going to throw in the towel and start pigging out again just because I slipped. I am not going to let this one screwup justify undoing everything I have worked so hard to accomplish.

I have told women time and again about the importance of standing up to adversity in their careers. I've talked about how easy it is to take cover and hide when storm clouds appear—as opposed to moving ahead despite the setbacks. I've repeated over and over how roadblocks in business are exhausting and can tempt you to give up—but that the key is to recognize them and know they can sabotage success. I've spoken at great length about how critical it is to keep going and never give up. No challenge is beyond us, because everything is figureoutable.

I think about standing, in a few months, on a huge stage in Austin in front of seven thousand cheering women because organizers of the annual Texas Conference for Women think I'm worth hearing. What a fraud I'd be if the truth is: *When it gets tough, Tory flees.* I owe it to myself, my family, and all the women I advise to regain my enthusiasm and determination and not beat myself up—as tempting as it is as I reflect on my sins of the past few days.

I hear my iPhone ping and it's an email from my friend Mindy in Orlando. As if by some sick coincidence, a cruel joke, she has picked this moment to let me know she has figured out who I remind her of: chubby Natalie on the 1980s sitcom *The Facts of Life.* It's been years since someone has told me this. As a teenager, I was horrified when classmates pointed out the similarity. Sure, Natalie had a healthy self-image and sharp wit, but if I longed to be compared to any character on that show, it was pretty Blair, not fat Natalie, no matter how confident she was. As a child, comments like this (*"She thinks I look like Natalie!"*) would have me making a beeline back to our snack-stuffed oven. In times of insult, embarrassment, pain, and panic, I always took cover with food.

But now, having made my Shift, familiar triggers are accompanied by big warning bells. I know that the smallest, most inconsequential things can set me off: a well-meaning friend or family member who says, "Come on, just this once." Off-limit foods served at special occasions like birthday parties, weddings, and holidays. A perceived insult, a bad day, or lousy weather. If there has been an excuse to eat, I have used it to always find my way to food—and the price I paid was staying fat. Those days are over.

In my desire to right my own ship, I look back to why I started on this journey in the first place. I envision sitting in the ABC cafeteria—waiting for Barbara to appear so I can break the news to her about the disaster in LA, when all I was trying to do was treat my daughter to a bit of fun.

"Okay, so you messed up?" I imagine Barbara saying as she approaches me.

Before I can respond, she says, "Big deal. Get going again. It's as simple as that."

I'm ready to put this Shift storm behind me and forge ahead. I'm resetting my clock and starting fresh—right now. Not tomorrow, not next week, and not at the beginning of the month. It's Day One, again.

Imagine this: someone who hasn't smoked in five months goes to a wedding, and before she knows it she's burned through five cigarettes with old friends. The next morning she buys a pack and within forty-eight hours she's started smoking again. A drinker quits for good on New Year's Day then finds herself at a Super Bowl party sipping a margarita. The next night she's back to three glasses of wine at dinner. If you're a foodie, a variation of this has no doubt played out for you at some point. Maybe you'll be at an event or out to dinner, or perhaps you'll just gorge yourself for the hell of it in the privacy of your own home. In any long-term struggle, you're bound to slip up and fall back to bad habits. It doesn't serve much purpose to beat yourself up. Resuming old ways will only hurt you more and leave you miserable. Accept that you, like everyone, are fallible, and there will be moments when you fall from grace—in your own eyes. When it happens, don't overthink it. Just wake up the very next day and start over again.

make the *Shift*

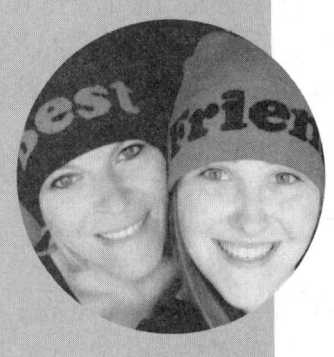

Remember what you loved to do as a kid: jump rope, swing a racket, roller-skate. Spend an afternoon revisiting a favorite activity.

Setbacks happen. Don't overthink them. Just start over immediately because each of us has the power to fix whatever's gone wrong.

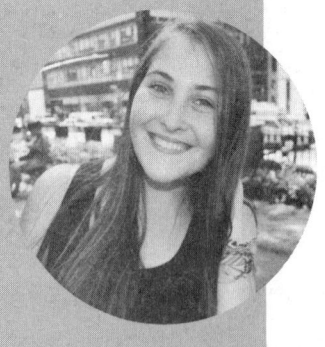

Listen to the fear, but don't let it paralyze you.

MONTH 9

The Dress

23

For many women, buying a dress is no big deal. But it has been almost three decades since I've worn one. In fact, I haven't put on a dress since a friend's bar mitzvah in 1983. In the throes of teenage puberty, I felt wildly self-conscious in my dowdy dress as I watched classmates on the dance floor showing off their cute bods in form-fitting numbers. I envied them more than I resented them. I would have loved to have been able to wear one of those short things—if I could be assured that people wouldn't laugh. Since that day, for dressy occasions, I've stuck to pants and a sweater, blouse, or blazer.

I've long disliked dressing rooms, given the enormous struggles with finding clothing that worked for me, yet now these are some of my favorite places. I am standing under lighting that's neither harsh nor soft enough to qualify as mood enhancing, while the saleswoman gets me a different size—a *smaller* one. I'd love to buy a dress for a wedding next week, an event that I have eagerly anticipated since the invitation arrived two months ago. Lara is one of my closest friends, and she and James are getting married in a vineyard on Long Island.

Over the summer I began to wonder whether I could risk wearing a dress there without looking ridiculous. When I casually mention it to Peter, he says without hesitation to go for it. "I predict you'll be pleasantly surprised."

After my six-pound weight gain on the trip with Emma, I worried about getting derailed long term. But I didn't. Instead, I immediately refocused, and once I was back on track, the pounds began to drop again, albeit slowly. An activity like shopping for new clothing proves that I'm genuinely making progress—not only in my mind, but around my waist too. I've always been a clotheshorse, but the old me shopped for stuff that would fit one too. Now, few things feel as good as watching my clothing size drop and experiencing the unique thrill that comes when you can fit into styles that had always been out of the question. I have new options now and I know every one of these choices will evaporate if I screw up. Knowing this motivates me to stay the course.

While I wait, I look at myself in the mirror. I place my right hand above my chest and slowly move it up. I'm touching the bone between my neck and shoulder. It's completely foreign to me—something I've not felt before. I have never even thought about my collarbone because I didn't know it was there: it had always been buried beneath layers of fat. Not only is fat disappearing from my body, but beautiful parts are emerging. I could get used to this.

For as long as I can remember, my profile resembled a female version of Alfred Hitchcock's famous pear-shaped cutout, with my belly extending past my boobs. But now as I turn sideways, I see that I've got an actual *figure* and that my breasts protrude over a flattened—not to be confused with *flat*—stomach. (Let's not get ahead of ourselves.) Incidentally, I don't have bee-sting boobs. They're more than ample C-cups, and I often bought 40C bras to be comfortable. Now, thanks to some melted back fat, my size has dropped to a 36.

Aside from my neck and boobs shrinking—and having a clear view of my toes when I look down—other parts of my body have also changed subtly. My fingers are leaner, and those teeny poofs of pinchable chubbiness between them have slowly disappeared and my rings need resizing. Snug shoes no longer hurt, and I can easily wear them all day without aching. My face is visibly thinner, enough so you can see my cheekbones when I talk. It's hardly gaunt, but it finally has natural definition—and not the kind created artificially by fancy contouring with blush and bronzer.

Before, in dressing rooms like this, I always faced full-length mirrors directly, not sideways, to avoid seeing the shelf that ran from my boobs to my waist. I was not *full*-figured, with discernible demarcations for chest, waist, and hips like a normal-sized woman. I was *no*-figured, with a brick body that ran from my double chin to my waist. Normally, I would be trying on something loose and blousy to hide my body, but today it's a fitted black dress in light wool. I'm assuming that Emma, who is trying on stuff in the next room, will be as candid as she always is when it comes to all things fashion.

The saleswoman returns with the dress: three-quarter sleeves, V-neck, tapered empire waist, and knee length—nothing resembling my standard uniform. When I put it on, I'm not only surprised but blown away, *stunned*, that the size 6 not only looks good but *great*.

"I think I could pull this off," I say out loud, fixated on myself in the mirror.

"What are you *doing*?" Emma says skeptically, inches away.

"Come in here," I say, pee-in-my-pants excited.

"I mean, Mom, you look *really good*. I've never seen you in a dress!" she says when she joins me seconds later and zips me up the last bit. "Dad will love it. *Buy* that sucker."

When Emma walks out, I morph into a self-centered, narcissistic teenager who can't get enough of herself in the mirror. I primp, pose, and pout, as if Justin Bieber is waiting for me and I want to look *hot*. I burst out laughing at how ridiculous this is: if there really *are* security personnel who monitor fitting rooms through hidden cameras and two-way mirrors, as I've always suspected, they must think they have a nut on their hands.

I can't wait to get home and model for Peter. I make him close his eyes and the look on his face when he opens them is so gratifying. Priceless.

"Sweetie, you look fantastic," he grins, giving me a kiss. "I can't wait to show off my skinny wife."

At the ceremony, I play with my wedding ring as we sit in white chairs next to rows of lush grapevines as Lara and James take their vows. I'm so happy that I'm wearing a dress because every woman here—save one—is too. I mention this to Peter as he manages to coax me onto the dance floor, where for the first time ever I get into the music, not worried at all about what others might think about my dance moves. I'm just another girl at the party, having fun. If I had worn pants I would have been the only woman who stood out— and not in a good way. That's always been my story line, but now having escaped that plight, I'm overcome with a sense of relief that's hard to fully describe. Not only are Peter and I honored to celebrate our friends' milestone in a classy setting where every detail is just right, but the night becomes one of our all-time favorites because of my newfound confidence. I'm not looking around comparing myself unfavorably to others. I'm not worried about dodging the party photographer for fear of him capturing unflattering shots. I'm not anxious to leave early. I am happy.

The morning after the wedding Emma waves her iPhone and suggests shooting selfies—photos of us together. "Me and hot Mama!"

"Hardly," I smile. "But I'm getting there."

Just then the phone rings, and as I talk outside the kitchen, I stare at our picture wall, a mix of framed photos of family and friends, plus a few of me posing with women at my events, that line the hallway to the kitchen.

I've always had an uneasy—at best—relationship with cameras based on many childhood shots of Fat Tory. Ever since, anyone taking my picture made me wary and anxious. I avoided cameras at parties and family events. If I couldn't, I tried to control the process as much as possible and sometimes went to embarrassing lengths, like grabbing the camera and taking photos of everyone *else*. At my conferences, attendees like to take photos with me as mementos, which I encourage and appreciate. But my terror at having "fat" photos circulating in cyberspace prompted me to take extraordinary measures. I'd ask women—in as lighthearted a way as possible—to not photograph me from below the stage looking up at an angle, "because if you do it'll show my double chin and I'll hate when it's posted on Facebook or Twitter." I was telling the truth, and invariably my plea was met with laughs from women in attendance who could relate. But a few times no one laughed, which made me want to run and hide. I stood on the stage and tried to be strong, even though I was quivering inside because I knew what some of them were thinking: *If I weighed as much as she does, photos would scare me too.*

Now, talking on the phone with Gianna from my office, I look at a photo of me with two women at a 2010 event in Los Angeles. I remember posting it on our wall because at the time I thought it was flattering. Now what I see is Fat Tory. I look at family shots: here I am hiding behind Peter and positioning my face just right (or so I think at the time) so it looks thin. Another shows me holding Jake and Emma as infants and wearing a jet-black turtleneck, which does its job: instead of seeing my fat neck, you see no neck. In photo after photo, I realize I have done *something* to hide how large I was. For years I actually thought I'd succeeded in making myself appear to be thin. I don't know who I was kidding, other than myself.

As I fill a cup of ice from the freezer, I cringe at my attempts to look "normal." I think for a split second about throwing away all the photos, but I know they're valuable reminders of who I never want to be again. I'll keep them just where they are and force myself to look whenever I'm even slightly tempted to return to bad habits. Some people use pictures from magazines or photos to visualize things they want or places they'd like to go. Images of a fancy car, an exotic vacation spot, or pricey jewelry motivate them to hustle. But for me the opposite works: while I want to run from the past, it serves a purpose—if only to remember how awful it was. My worst pictures, the ones I'd typically tear up or delete, are powerful visual tools to keep me moving forward, in the right direction. I don't ever want to look that way again, and no pizza, pasta, or pie is worth risking a return to those dark days.

"Come on, Mom!" Emma yells from her room, where she has been waiting for me since Gianna called. I'm actually looking forward to this because I've become much more comfortable with cameras.

"Here I am," I say in her doorway, and we get down to business. She grabs her iPhone again and we pose like supermodels, with Emma extending her hand to shoot photos of us at different angles. She clicks dozens of times. We alternately smile with teeth and without, serious, laughing, and sucking in our cheeks then blowing them out. We're having a great time and I'm no longer sweating every shot. Of course I want to look good, but I'm not concerned about appearing huge because I'm not anymore. Little moments like this inspire me to keep going.

A New Kind of Birthday Celebration

24

We celebrated my forty-second birthday last night with a group of friends and family. We had planned to take everyone on one of our favorite New York things to do—a Circle Line cruise around Manhattan—but the weather looked sketchy. So instead we had a Greek feast at our apartment. Knowing everyone would expect a birthday cake, we had one, but planned another sweet for me. After nine months and a nearly fifty-pound weight loss, I am at a point where I am confident in my ability to resist overindulgence: I'm ready to handle sweets. Definitely not birthday cake, just the right ones in moderation, perhaps once a week or so, not every day.

I've discovered two delicious, guilt-free treats. Hail Merry chocolate macaroons each have sixty-five calories and five carbs and are made from organic maple syrup, shredded coconut, dark cocoa, Madagascar bourbon vanilla, and sea salt. They taste as good as Godiva—better, actually. As do Sweetriot cacao nibs, which are covered in 70 percent dark chocolate. The nibs are smaller than a chocolate chip, about the size of a Tic Tac, and come in tins. These treats are just two calories each and pack a huge punch for their tiny size. That night, while everyone else enjoys the cake, a macaroon and a few nibs do the trick for me.

A little while after the guests left, Peter handed me a ring box, and inside was a super-thin diamond band. "I love the slimmer you," his note read. "But I love the more confident and happier you even more."

Now three quarters of the way through the year that is changing my life, I am realizing what the Shift is doing to my inner self. By being a little selfish, I have become a lot happier. This, in turn, upped the happiness of everyone around me: Peter, my kids, my staff. In her bestseller *The Happiness Project*, author Gretchen Rubin writes, "One of the most enduring myths about happiness is that it's selfish to try to be happier." All of the studies show, as I myself have discovered this year, that happier people are more generous, better leaders, and have stronger social bonds. When we're unhappy, we turn inward. Happiness actually makes us turn outward and think more about the world around us. It's for this reason that Gretchen, who has shared her message at my Spark & Hustle events, says, "We should be selfish, if only for selfless reasons." I would paraphrase that to say, "You should Shift, first for yourself, then to benefit everyone you love."

"Do I See a Slimmer Tory Johnson?"

uring a live *GMA* segment on September 21, a date I'll never forget, an off-the-cuff comment by Sam Champion reinforces that I'm on the right track and will look like a fool if I mess up. It's a crisp fall morning and a large crowd has gathered with their signs outside the Times Square studio. I've dressed in a Lafayette 148 black silk button-down top and tight black jeans, and I'm about four inches taller than usual, thanks to sky-high Stuart Weitzman platform wedges. I'm doing my segment with Elizabeth Vargas, who is filling in for Robin Roberts as she recovers from her bone marrow transplant. The last "Deals & Steals" offering on my table display is a selection of oversized men's watches. As I'm wrapping up, Sam pops into frame and slides one of them onto his wrist. "Do I see a slimmer Tory Johnson?" he blurts out on live TV. I want to crawl under the table. I'm praying the camera cuts away. But Sam continues: "You look terrific!"

I spontaneously hand him all of the watches, as if bribing him for his compliments—or to zip it. When we finally go to commercial, Sam hugs me and says, "I don't know if it's deliberate or accidental, but you've lost a lot and look fantastic." We smile for photos, one of which I post on Facebook. Within minutes I am flooded with emails, Facebook comments, and tweets asking for my secret: "Sam's right: You do look terrific." "Tory, you're melting away." "Tell us how you've done it."

The positive feedback makes my day. At first when people commented on my shrinking frame, I was embarrassed, humiliated, and slightly frightened by the unsolicited attention: I could only guess at what they *used* to think about my body but were polite enough not to say. But now, since I like my new self much more, my appreciation for their kind words has shot up, way up. You've got to *embrace encouragement*, and besides, who among us doesn't like to be told we're looking good—especially after we've worked so hard to change? In any difficult journey you have to stop frequently and look at what is going right. Use compliments to inspire and motivate—not as permission slips to stop or revert to old ways.

Until this moment, I had shied away from even talking about my weight or new routine privately, let alone publicly on national TV. This had always been my personal battle and

I wanted it to stay that way. But after all the poignant feedback I begin to get from women who commented on the picture of Sam and me, plus dozens and dozens of emails, it reminds me how weight is also an ongoing, silent struggle for millions of women. For years, I have used my platform on TV to help women get hired, start businesses, and save money. Why couldn't I share my lifelong weight battle—and the steps I took to conquer it—to help them do it too? That night I decide to write this book.

I've always enjoyed working with women to help them get ahead in their careers, whether it's through advice in books, articles, or speeches; at events; or even on the phone. And over the years I have become an expert on how to find a job and succeed in the world of small business. But no advice I have ever given to anyone resonates inside me as much as this subject. I also have a selfish motive in writing about my weight struggles: I think it will keep me honest and inspire me to live healthy. Who in her right mind would write a book about losing a lot of weight—then gain it all back again? Not I, that's for sure.

I realize that I can't let my current giddiness and success derail my progress. That's what I always did when I lost a bit of weight. I'd get to a certain benchmark and feel a need to reward myself for reaching it. Why did I feel a need to pat myself on the back? Because it's a favorite theme with diet gurus who preach that the way to stay motivated is to *reward yourself* when you are good. Many of them say the best way to do it is with a sinful meal—and maybe it works for some people, but it never did for me. I couldn't understand how Jared lost all that weight eating nothing but Subway sandwiches. We've all read about the woman who lost a hundred pounds on one of these diets—any diet—saying the only way she could stay sane was by eating pizza a couple times a week. Pizza! God bless her if it worked, but I think people who succeed on plans like that are the rare exception. Cheat meals and the like were the kinds of things I did routinely and they always derailed me: I'd cheer myself for losing ten pounds with a "hard-earned" indulgent meal followed by dessert—and within days I'd be eating with abandon again. *Rewarding myself, a recovering food addict, with food is akin to an alcoholic celebrating a month of sobriety with a beer or two. It doesn't work.*

With the Shift, there is no end to celebrate because this is a lifetime *deal. I must not only watch what I eat and how much I exercise for the long haul, but also be conscious about staying motivated.* My initial impetus for losing weight was my real fear of getting fired from *GMA*. But with time I've moved away from that worry. Encouraging emails and "Attagirl!" comments from *GMA* colleagues and viewers have boosted my confidence big-time. I know that I can't kick back: I must find new sources of inspiration wherever I can.

I review the journals I kept sporadically over the years, particularly entries where I talk about the joy that certain milestones and moments brought me. How I was determined to lead a long, happy, and fun life. I look back at what I wrote about Emma and Jake learning to walk and the drive that ended with us buying the country house. But I also look at entries I wrote about how miserable and unhappy I was with my size—and how I lacked the willpower to do anything about it, which troubled me. *When am I ever going to deal with this?* I wrote in July 1999, after returning home depressed from a party at a beach club where every woman wore a sleeveless dress except me. *I will never go to another event again and be the fat girl,* I wrote in an entry in 2008 after participating in a women's conference. *How am I going to make sure that Emma doesn't end up obese like me?* asks an entry in 2010. There are so many passages like these, sad to say, and I go back and review them all. They remind me that I don't ever want to relive those days. Never again.

make the *Shift*

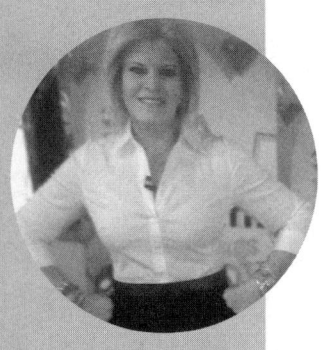

Rewarding myself, a recovering food addict, with food is akin to an alcoholic celebrating a month of sobriety with a beer or two. It doesn't work.

With the Shift, there is no end to celebrate because this is a lifetime deal.

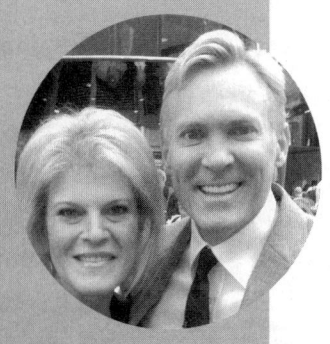

MONTH 10

26

Johnson Family Fun Nights

"**M**ove like Jagger!" Emma shouts. "Faster, faster, Mama! Let's go!"

If she puts her heart in it, I think Em could be a backup dancer for any pop star. I marvel at her coordination and effortless rhythm since I spent most of my life shying away from dance floors. At first I am skeptical when she proposes these dancing sessions, but I've come to love it when we meet in her room and move our asses to a playlist that includes ten of our faves, like "Sexy and I Know It" by LMFAO; "Dynamite" by Taio Cruz; "Whistle" by Flo Rida; "Dance Again" by J.Lo, featuring Pitbull; "Single Ladies" by Beyoncé; "Forget You" by Cee Lo Green; and "Firework" by Katy Perry.

We don't stop until the music does—thirty minutes of insanity. Emma makes sure there's no downtime. It's an ongoing booty shake a few nights a week in our house.

Jason Derulo's "Ridin' Solo" is blaring from an iPod speaker on Emma's desk and we're belting out the lyrics and dancing like wild in what has become one of my favorite rituals. I love letting loose—behind closed doors—as if we are in the middle of the craziest dance floor of the hottest nightclub on New Year's Eve. I feel great when we're done. Dancing relieves some stress of my day and I find that afterward I'm not as hungry. Or maybe I am but not about to let that action go to waste by shoveling down a big dinner.

Exercise is still an issue for me. I wish I could say that I was at the point where I could do a full-on aerobic workout or even a decent intense jog on the treadmill, but my hatred of breaking a sweat runs deep. Not being very physically coordinated probably has something to do with it. Even after all these years, at heart I'm still the girl who forged a doctor's note to get out of high school gym class. When I couldn't avoid PE, teachers forced me to do activities I often failed at spectacularly—everyone has seen the fat kid founder in gym class—so I have a lifelong fear of exercise to overcome, and old habits die hard for this couch potato. I keep telling myself: *One step at a time, serious exercise will come.*

My other favorite evening activity comes on Friday when we celebrate the end of the week with Johnson Family Fun Night. Pre-Shift, Peter, Jake, Emma, and I would indulge in a high-calorie meal at a favorite restaurant. That had to go, but instead of abandoning our ritual, we found new ways to spend this time together. We bowl or hit the batting cages. There's mini golf on nearby Randall's Island. We walk the popular High Line, a mile-long elevated path on Manhattan's West Side that once served as a railroad. Every once in a while, we take a twilight cruise like tourists around the city on the Circle Line.

I take a quick shower after tonight's dance craze. Peter serves us a chopped salad for dinner, filled with a medley of brightly colored fresh vegetables. For dessert, I have a small bowl of berries, which is a big deal as it's the most fruit I've had in months. As a native of the Sunshine State, I love fruit but have so far avoided it, seeing as an apple has the equivalent of my entire daily carb ration. Now I decide that I can reintroduce berries a couple times a week—not a huge bowl, but a small handful of blueberries, raspberries, blackberries, or strawberries. For the first time ever, I find them yummier than cupcakes: *Sacrifice can be sweet.*

The Treadmill Is Not My Enemy

arly in the year I was red-faced and winded when the elevator broke, forcing me to walk four flights to our office several times in one day. It was a stark reminder, not that I needed one, that I needed to figure out this whole fitness thing. Slowly I have incorporated bits of movement into my daily routine five days a week. I walk to and from my office, a thirty-block, one-and-a-half-mile stroll. I make a point of getting up at lunchtime and doing *some* errand in the afternoon—anything—so that I don't sit on my butt all day. I even stop cruising around for a parking space to open up near mall entrances. Instead, I park wherever I find the first opening and hoof it. And I embraced the outdoors over the summer in the country. I know: none of it would impress a jock, but it's something.

I owe some of these baby steps to my colleague Alex, who is a fitness buff. We've had an all-day meeting in Boston and are heading back to New York on the Acela. A few minutes before the high-speed train pulls away from Back Bay Station, we stop at a newsstand to buy magazines, bottled water, and nuts to snack on.

"You're so good," Alex says.

She sees that I have resisted an assortment of chips and junk food, a far cry from my former travel routine when she'd watch me grab cheesy Smartfood popcorn, Rold Gold pretzels, or a Kit Kat bar for a ride on a train, plane, or automobile. Alex knows firsthand how hard I work on food choices, but she also senses that exercise continues to be a struggle for me.

"So how's it going with working out?" she asks, as we settle into our seats.

"I want to do more and I know I need to do more, but I'm just stuck," I say, defeated.

Alex is sympathetic. "I know a lot of people who want to get in shape and vow to spend an hour a day on the treadmill," she says. "But it's very easy to say no when you're staring at a sixty-minute workout. It's daunting."

"For sure," I say. "But what's the alternative?"

"Don't start with an hour in mind, because you'll give up before you even get going. You'll be 'too busy' or just not that into it," she says. "Telling yourself you'll walk for five or even ten minutes isn't so scary. If you can commit to as little as five minutes, you'll find yourself increasing to twenty and then thirty minutes, and you can build from there. The key is to just start. Anything is better than nothing."

"Five minutes is a number I can relate to," I tell her. "If my producers are feeling generous with airtime, it's just slightly more than the length of one of my TV segments."

"Then start with that," Alex says.

Her advice makes sense and feels manageable. In the past, similar conversations would have left me thinking, *Yes, but . . .*, as I tried any which way to change the topic. This time *I'm encouraged rather than intimidated*—a good sign. Besides, I need something to push me forward to my next weight milestone, and a regular exercise regimen could help kick-start me to the next level. If there's one thing I'm ready for, it's to lose more, faster.

When I arrive home that night, I ride up in the elevator with Leesa, my next-door neighbor who always wears sleek exercise outfits. Tonight is no different.

"You're disappearing before our very eyes," she whispers to me. She's a beautiful, stay-at-home mom who devotes a chunk of her day to working out at the gym and she has a tight, thin body. For years, as someone with a busy career, I dismissed her obsession with exercise, chalking it up to her being a lady of leisure. *What else does she have to do?* But now that I value my changing body, I've come to view Leesa and other yoga-, spin-, and Pilates-fixated women in workout wear in a new light: they have adopted lifelong habits that ensure their health and fitness, not just physically but mentally too. What's not to like and admire about that? Leesa *cares* about her body image and *works* at it every single day and that's a *good* thing, not something that deserves scorn, which I no doubt felt before out of petty jealousy.

"One of these days I'll join you at the gym," I tell her.

"Anytime!" she says, and she means it.

My brother, David, has always given me diet tips but has now progressed to passionate lobbying regarding exercise equipment. He is determined to get me to fall in love with one of his favorites: a cross-country ski machine.

Although he claims he has to work hard to keep his thirty-two-inch waist, I also think he got good thin genes along with natural discipline. He's a tall, lean hottie, my brother, with no body fat. So when I tell him I am finally interested in some fitness equipment that I can use at home (I'm still not ready to brave a gym), he is eager to help and sends me an evangelical message about the NordicTrack. "You're going to love it. It's so easy." He continues to sing its praises incessantly until he finally comes up with the magic words: "It'll give you a full-body workout in just twenty minutes." I like the sound of that: less time than an episode of *Jeopardy!*

"You'll never use it. Guaranteed," Peter says, doubtful. He explains that as a kid in upstate New York, he and his friends used to cross-country ski and that it was one of the most exhausting things he's ever done. "I know you and this is not for you."

But I am determined. "My brother knows me too. And he thinks it would be great for me," I say. "I want to at least give it try."

That weekend, Peter surprises me with a barely used Nordic-Track that he scored for a bargain at the flea market downtown.

After lugging the thing upstairs and setting it up next to our bed, the only available spot in our apartment, Peter says, "I appreciate your initiative, baby. Maybe you'll get into it."

"But you still don't think I'll use it, do you?"

"Love you," he says, changing the subject.

I'm determined to use it, if anything to prove him wrong. That week, I ski in our bedroom three, maybe four times. But never for more than ten minutes. It's exhausting, just as Peter said it would be. I am ready to give up. Peter gets on it maybe a dozen times, then gives it to our doorman after Palmer says he wants to get in shape. (A few weeks later on our way out the door, there's the machine, curbside, waiting for the garbage pickup. Guess Palmer didn't like it either.)

I consult with David again, and this time he suggests an elliptical, which he and my sister-in-law Julie are hooked on. "It not only works your legs but your arms too. Full body. Perfect for you."

"Not this again," Peter says skeptically as we head over the George Washington Bridge in search of yard sales that I found promoted on Craigslist. "Do me a favor. This time before we buy a machine, will you spend a few minutes on it to see if you like it?"

"Deal."

I am already ahead of him and have worn a black tracksuit for the occasion.

I find one at the home of a woman who tells me that she used to do personal training out of her garage but now trains at the local gym. Hence her need to get rid of the equipment. She even arranges to have someone deliver it to our home for an extra hundred bucks. I am sold.

I use the elliptical twice as much as the NordicTrack—at least eight times—and each time I collapse red-faced after just a few minutes. I come to hate this computerized version of a medieval torture rack. Better for clothes, I think, and they soon hang from it.

"Hey, Palmer, I got another machine if you want it," Peter says to him in our lobby.

"That's okay," Palmer responds with a wink.

"What the hell?" Peter shouts a few days later, stumbling over a box that someone has left inside the front door, a twenty-pound square that does not move when his foot hits it.

"Oh, those must be the kettlebells from David," I say.

"Use these every day and you'll have abs of steel," reads David's note tucked inside. He is unrelenting, not only foisting exercise *ideas* on me but now exercise *gifts* too. Clearly he won't stop until something clicks. That evening he comes over to our apartment and leads me through a series of moves with the heavy bells in our living room. It seems easy enough, but it requires me to actually do it when David is not there to monitor me. I'm always eager to give new things a try, then even more eager to abandon them in record time.

After a few solo attempts, I decide that dancing with Emma is easier and a hell of a lot more fun. And so it goes: the kettlebells become first-rate doorstops and Peter takes control of this madness, goes to a sporting goods store and buys a standard treadmill—our fourth piece of exercise equipment in almost as many weeks.

"A treadmill is different," Peter tells me the next morning after he makes an inaugural run on it. "It's easy and there's really no excuse for not getting on it every day. You don't have to run. You can just walk while you watch TV, listen to music, or talk to Emma."

"Whatever, baby," I say, returning to a Page Six item in the *New York Post* about Kim Kardashian and Kanye West house hunting in Miami. Must be a slow news day.

Peter leaves the room to take a shower. After seeing how little effort it took for him to get moving on the machine and thinking endlessly about my chat with Alex, I decide to hop on the damn thing myself. I'll do it for eight minutes—a compromise between her suggested five and ten. Nothing impressive, but light-years from what I would normally do, which is nothing. If I do this in the morning and then dance with Emma at night, I think, it just might count as a full workout.

Eventually—over weeks, not days—I work myself up to a fast walk for thirty minutes on the treadmill several times a week. As I increase the time I make a pact with myself: I can only add minutes, not subtract them. I set the speed between four and four and a half miles an hour, which means thirty minutes gets me at least a two-mile walk. There's no marathon in my future, but I keep telling myself that every bit counts—and it does. With each turn, the treadmill becomes more palatable and just something I *do*. I watch TV as I walk, and when it becomes tiring or challenging, I purposely daydream about something I have coming up or funny things Peter and the kids have said—anything to get my mind off the task at hand. The point is I am doing it.

make the *Shift*

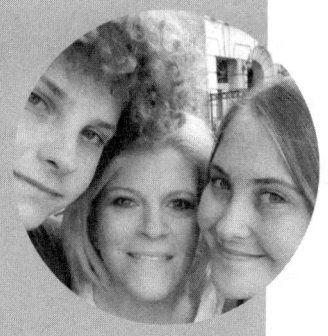

When it comes to exercise, start with anything, because it's better than nothing. Look to be inspired, not intimidated, until you find the workout that works best for you.

Sacrifice can be sweet. Pass the berries!

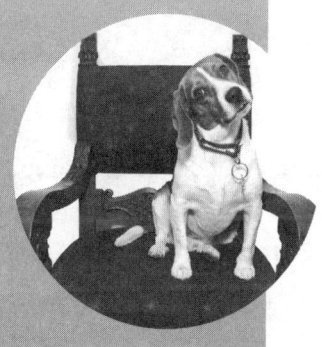

MONTH 11

28

. . . So Much to Be Thankful For

G rowing confidence in my body has translated not only into a happier Tory but also a hotter Tory, at least in bed. After what has become a frequent morning romp, Peter and I begin discussing the logistics of daily life. Today, it's about Thanksgiving. Good-bye, hot mama; hello, *Modern Family*. It's not quite as sexy, but with two dozen guests descending on us next week, planning is a must.

I was initially nervous about this holiday, but an unexpected request for me to appear live on *GMA* on Thanksgiving morning could be my saving grace. Usually, all of us would be at the country house cooking dinner for the friends and family who'll join us Thursday. I would have consumed two thousand calories just doing taste tests while making standard side dishes like corn bread stuffing with sage, sausage, and roasted chestnuts; green bean casserole topped with those scrumptious, high-carb crispy onions; and fully-loaded macaroni and cheese. But this year, Peter and the kids drive to the country Wednesday night without me and begin to handle the preparations, while I stay home in Manhattan for the TV segment.

I get to the house midmorning on Thanksgiving and everything is done and ready to go, with competing aromas of fried bacon, roast turkey, and various scented candles that Emma has lit. I take a deep breath and soak it all in, then make a mental affirmation that I will not overeat—a promise I intend to keep. *Just eat sensibly*, I say to myself, and I do a few hours later when everyone arrives.

I stick to turkey, salad, and some of my sister-in-law Kate's sugar-free lime Jell-O with walnuts, diced apples, and bits of chopped celery. It's a perfect combination of tang and crunch. I watch everyone else take seconds—even thirds—of all the dishes we've laid out, but I've prepared myself for this day and I'm neither tempted nor jealous. Let them feast, I think, while I enjoy my choices too. In past years, trying to "be good" at Thanksgiving would have made me miserable and, probably to some extent, my family too. Who wants a moody dieter during a holiday feast? But I'm no longer concerned with being good or bad because that's not what the Shift is all about.

Instead, I'm disciplined enough to know what I normally eat and I stick to it. While Thanksgiving remains a special day in terms of food, it's just another Thursday for me with choices to make. It is not a big deal because I choose to make it this way. Yes, our home is filled with many more options than usual, but so what? Just because it's there doesn't mean I must touch it. Several months ago, I would have felt like I was missing out, but now I am at peace with my reality.

That night after everyone's gone, the dishwasher is running, and the kids are asleep downstairs, Peter and I sit in bed and do our postmortem on the day, chatting about the relatives we only see a few times a year and what they had to say.

Out of the blue, Peter says, "I was impressed by your restraint."

"Huh?" I ask, not sure what he means.

"I'm talking about what you ate," he says.

"You hadn't noticed any of my restraint until now?"

"Of course, but today you seemed to take it to a new level. Everyone was gorging themselves, and you ignored it all," he says. "And you didn't seem out of sorts about it."

"I kept thinking how much I'd regret it if I overindulged even on a holiday that revolves around food," I say. "It wasn't worth ruining the day by going on carbo-load."

Pointing to his stomach, Peter says, "I hear you on that. I think I enjoyed a bit too much."

"Plus, I *did* indulge. I tasted David and Julie's brownies

and shared an oatmeal chocolate chip cookie with Emma," I
admit. "Avoiding the two pumpkin pies wasn't hard because
I'm not into pumpkin pie. And yes, I did keep myself busy all
day, which distracted me from thinking about all the food
that was around here."

Peter asks me about restraint—of how I got to the point
where a taste of a brownie is enough, when normally I'd eat
four of them.

"I have to keep telling myself that the momentary satisfac-
tion I would get while scarfing down a tray of warm brownies isn't worth the misery I'll feel tomorrow when I get on the
scale and see the repercussions of my gluttony," I say. "A bite
won't hurt me, as long as that's where it stops. But overindulgence is what did me in, and I'm not falling back into that."

"Doesn't it feel great to defeat something that has always
beaten you?" Peter asks.

"Better than anything."

"Anything?" he smiles, while pulling me closer and slipping his hand down my pants.

On our drive back to the city the next afternoon, I think
about this conversation and how Peter was not only impressed
with how far I've come but, in a way, grateful too. Not grateful that *he* is no longer saddled with a fat wife, but grateful
that *I* am no longer burdened by my weight. He's happy that
I no longer allow weight problems to torment *me*.

I've always *acted* confident, and I think most people who
know me would say that of all my shortcomings, a lack of

confidence was not one of them. But I knew better. *I took pains to hide my vulnerability, terrified what people would think if they knew that the real Tory defined herself mentally not as a smart woman but simply a fat one.* Beneath the outwardly self-assured me was a woman who worked desperately hard to mask her weakness.

MONTH 12

29

Hello, World

With each passing week, I get more and more notes from viewers cheering me on. Far from cringing when women mention my weight loss, I embrace their stories and assure them that they can do it too. I feel myself bonding with them on a defining issue of our lives. Helping women further their careers or venture out on their own has been extremely satisfying professionally and always warmed my heart. But bonding on an issue that tarred me for so long is so much more personally satisfying. I'm touched that women I've never met feel comfortable enough to talk to me about such a personal struggle. Women like Donna in

New Jersey, who described herself in an email as "an unem-
ployed, happy, hot flash wife and mom."

"This all started when I lost my job two years ago. I'm
having such a hard time trying to get in shape and lose
weight. I'm a stress eater and I hate to work out, oh yes, and
I'm in full-blown menopause. Uhh!"

There was a time when I had enough difficulty simply
dealing with my own weight issues, let alone others'. When
women would email me and ask how I was losing weight, I
was too embarrassed to answer. Me, talk about my "weight
problem"? No chance. But now, I'm all ears, and instead of
ignoring their emails, I write back to encourage them.

I know it's hard and I ask what has and hasn't worked—
and why? More often than not, we wind up agreeing that it's
not the diets themselves that don't work, but that we gave up
too soon and our heads weren't really into it. I tell them I had
to get to a point where the only thing that finally clicked was
a combination of fear and being fed up—and making a fundamental Shift with a clarity and determination that I had
never mustered before. Invariably, they get that instantly,
and I encourage them all to tap into that disgust and keep it
close.

I've met women I never would have guessed could have
struggled with anything, let alone their weight. I discover
that my colleague at WABC, meteorologist Amy Freeze and
her husband won $100,000 in the 1999 Body-for-Life fit-
ness contest. Discouraged by her inability to lose weight after the birth of their son, Amy and Gary partnered for the

twelve-week program and together lost forty-eight pounds of fat and gained twenty pounds of muscle.

"One of the great lessons of life is using your mind to alter your body and then having that physical transition alter your philosophy on your individual potential," she says.

Amy says losing weight allowed her to see the power she had to change her body. "It's very liberating to alter your physique, and it makes you believe that you can change anything about yourself, that there are no limits in life."

What she says resonates so strongly inside me, having spent my entire life truly believing that I was doomed to be trapped forever in a body I didn't like.

A couple weeks into December, and it's so cold that I need a coat for an outdoor segment on *GMA*. Just two months earlier I had my favorite long black suede coat altered: the tailor overhauled the arms, shoulders, and waist, so much so that he joked we could make another jacket with the leftover material.

But today, the first time I've worn it since it was fixed, the jacket feels too big. Evelyn Mason, *GMA*'s head stylist, has a solution: she pulls out big metal clamps—binder clips for stacks of paper too big to staple. As I face the mirror in her wardrobe room, she stands behind me and pulls the fabric to add definition to my waist and tightens the loose material above and below it. With six clamps firmly in place on the back of my coat, my shapely silhouette appears.

"You're getting smaller every time I see you." Evelyn smiles.

"And you, even sweeter," I say, returning her grin.

When I head outside, a woman in the crowd sees the clips on my back and jokes that I look like a portable office supply closet. She's impressed with my little trick.

The Perfect Moment Is Now

30

A winter coat tailored with binder clips is the last thing I need when we head to sunny Miami Beach for Christmas week. We haven't spent the holidays there in a few years, opting instead for road trips. This year David, Julie, and Charlotte will also be staying at my parents' house, along with Emma and Jake. Peter and I opt to check into a hotel in South Beach to make it feel more like a private getaway for us. We take long morning walks on the beach, something I never did as a child, and spend hours sitting by the pool talking and reading. The kids join us a few afternoons, and we have big family dinners each night.

After a meal at a Spanish restaurant in Aventura, Mom pulls me aside as we walk to our car.

"I am so proud of you. You look so good. I wish I had your strength," she says.

"You do," I respond. "You just haven't tapped into it yet."

This is not a new conversation for either of us. For months now, practically every time she sees me on TV, Mom has called, emailed, or texted to say how good I look and how proud she is. But the truth is she has always praised me. If there were Olympic medals for Moms Who Cheer Their Kids On, she would win gold. She's as generous as they come. I've always looked good in her eyes. But I also know that weight is a touchy topic for her—because she can't get a handle on hers—so we don't get into deep discussions about it, and when the subject comes up we stick to superficial chitchat. I can't push someone who isn't ready, and with Mom I have found that it's always "yes, but . . ." The latest is that she is stressed because my grandmother was diagnosed with Alzheimer's earlier in the year and the burden of her care is falling largely on my mother. Even though Grandma has round-the-clock, live-in help, my mother worries about her nonstop. She's the caring daughter who can't help herself. Obviously, Mom has a lot on her mind, and in many ways I can easily see why this illness is a legitimate excuse for her to go easy on herself.

When I think back on it now, I too leaned on excuses for years. I'd tell myself, sure, I want to be thin, but I'm too down after being fired from a job I loved. Yes, I'd like to lose weight, but Peter's newspaper career ended, and now our family relies on *me* for full financial support, so I can't focus on a diet right now. Of course I'd like to eat better, but the stress of getting my kids through the archaic, tortuous process of transitioning from middle school to high school in New York City prevents me from tackling my health right now. Yada yada.

The list, if I think about it, was as endless for me as it is for anyone who is looking for a "yes, but . . ." way out. *There will always be curveballs thrown your way, which you can either deflect or let hit you right in the gut—and take you out of the game.* But one thing is consistent no matter how many stressors we all face: we *choose* what we put in our mouths. I can't force Mom to follow my plan—so I'm not going to become the nagging daughter who harasses her to get with the program. She knows I'm here to help when she decides the time is right and announces that she's ready. I'm hopeful that day will come for her.

It reminds me of a lesson I learned years ago, when Jake and Emma were in preschool at the YMCA in our neighborhood and became friends with a cute kid named Michael whose mom happened to be Kelly Ripa. The kids became friends and Kelly and I did too.

If you've ever watched *Live*, you know the show begins with several minutes of host chat on everything from major current events to what they had for dinner last night. So at one point very early in our friendship, I told Peter I wanted to ask Kelly to talk about an upcoming women's conference I was hosting. "Great," he said, "do it." I told myself I'd ask her the next time we were together. But each time our kids played at school, the park, or one of our apartments, I chickened out. I kept telling myself I'd do it when "the time was right." In retrospect, I was waiting for the perfect moment, something I couldn't define. What conditions constitute the right time for anything? I said I'd know it when I felt it, as if I were waiting for celestial birds to chirp around my head or for Kelly to intuit via osmosis that I had something on my mind—without me saying a word to her. After a month of stalling, my event was now just a week away. Peter told me that unless I stopped practicing my little pitch to Kelly in front of the mirror and actually talked to her, he was going to do it himself. So I did it that day and Kelly said sure, of course, no problem. Done. The next day she and her cohost at the time, Regis Philbin, chatted on-air about my event. I learned then that waiting for the perfect time is a waste of time because it just delays action.

Whenever I catch myself stalling or avoiding uncomfortable things, I remind myself of that day. It's as relevant now as it was then. *Instead of focusing on excuses, I envision results.* I hope Mom can do this someday.

On our last day in Miami, I get an email from Barbara asking where I'm staying because she's seen me tweet that I'm in South Beach. It turns out we're at adjacent hotels, and we agree to meet at her pool for a quick hello. The thought of seeing her—even for a few minutes—makes me anxious. I've bumped into her only a couple of times in the last several months, but in the back of my mind I wonder: When she sees me now, will she think I look as good as *I* think I do? Or will she walk away disappointed? *Tory still has a very long way to go.*

She immediately puts all my worries to rest with a big, warm hug. She tells me how happy she is for me and how great I look. I'll never forget the first email she sent me in March— the one that said "You are looking fantastic"—and how thrilled I was to get it. Barbara launches right into an admission: she thought I hated her after our morning in the cafeteria. Peter interrupts and begins teasing her, saying I spent the year throwing darts at an oversized poster of her photo in our bedroom. That gets all of us laughing. We talk about how it all played out, and Barbara tells me that she's amazed that I actually *did* something.

"Why?" I ask.

"Because I've had similar talks with other people and their reactions are far different. They don't see what I see. They don't see an opportunity for change or improvement. Or they're convinced everything is just fine. It all boils down to them not being open to hearing whatever 'it' is that I see," she explains. Her husband, Andrew, nods knowingly, having heard it all before.

"But aren't they worried about losing their jobs, like I was about mine?" I ask.

No way, she says, and she tells me pointedly that my on-air role was never in jeopardy. That comes as both a relief and surprise.

"I know you never threatened me but I still marvel at how

smoothly you delivered the message without ever dangling the possibility of a pink slip," I tell her. "I always assumed that I'd be out if I didn't shape up—literally."

"We love you and we've always loved you," Barbara says. I can't help but wonder if that's more tactful than truthful, but welcome words to me nonetheless.

(Incidentally, remember Sandy the stylist Barbara offered to connect me with during the Conversation? I never heard another word about that proposal, which to me confirmed what I suspected from the beginning: This was not about my hair or clothes. It was about my weight—and that's a good thing, because focusing on attire would have been yet another gimmick that ignored the real issue.)

On our flight back to New York that afternoon, I think about how satisfying it was to hear Barbara's positive and encouraging words, which make what I've accomplished this year feel so much sweeter. After all, just a year earlier, I was about as heavy as I'd ever been, fed up with the way I looked, and just beginning to come to grips with the long slog ahead. To know that I actually *did something*, that I *turned my life around* in the course of exactly one year, is as satisfying as anything I've ever experienced.

This gets me thinking about a story a few months earlier that struck a chord nationally because it dealt with two hot-button issues: obesity and bullying. At a local TV station in La Crosse, Wisconsin, veteran anchor Jennifer Livingston went on-air to stand up for herself after she got a fat-shaming email from a viewer. "The truth is I *am* overweight," Livingston said. "You can call me fat, even obese on a doctor's chart. Do you think I don't know that? You're not a friend of mine. You're not part of my family ... You know nothing about me that you don't see on the outside. I am much more than a number on a scale."

But the tone of the writer's email, Livingston said, angered her even more than the comments about her weight. The man who wrote it said he never intended to bully her, but Livingston perceived it that way. She said bullying is something that kids and parents should recognize and fight. "This behavior is learned. It is passed down. If you're at home and you're talking about the fat news lady, guess what, your children are probably going to go to school and call someone fat."

"Good for her!" Peter and I said in unison at the time, when we saw her on *GMA*. Over the course of almost seven years at *GMA*, I've gotten only a handful of messages from viewers about my weight, but the sting was equivalent to hearing from millions of people. They encouraged me to try the weight-loss shakes they were peddling, suggested wearing bigger jewelry more proportional to my size, and a few just spit it out and told me to lose weight. I hit "delete" on all their emails and ignored their advice.

Now, I think about how Livingston was positioned as a hero for loving herself as she is. I admire her for that. She seemed genuine and I was happy to see someone on TV take a stand against society's obsessive fixation on body image and thinness. But part of me recognized in her the *old* Tory, who was not ready to deal with some very real consequences of being obese.

I could have easily been outraged that Barbara dared to speak up. Just as I always was when well-meaning viewers gave me unsolicited advice. The truth is *I was ready to hear Barbara's message*, so much so that all she had to do was *hint* at the real issue. I took it from there. Instead of viewing Barbara as the heavy, I looked at her as a savior. For the first time ever, I was open to help. *I was ready to make the Shift.*

Barbara saved me from myself, from me continuing to think that it was my destiny to live in a body I never liked and that I had no options. In the span of just a few minutes, she helped me move to a whole new place in life. Since that day, Barbara has become my personal weight-loss whisperer, continuing to send me little notes telling me how happy she is—for me. Our little talk continues to fuel my success. Hell, even Scott's nitpicking motivates me, if only to prove him wrong. As the pounds continue to come off—slowly, surely, and for good—I know that I'm not grieving for the fat girl I once was. I accept who I was and the size I was for the first forty years of my life, and I've worked hard to move toward the woman I want to be for the rest of my life. There's no turning back now.

make the *Shift*

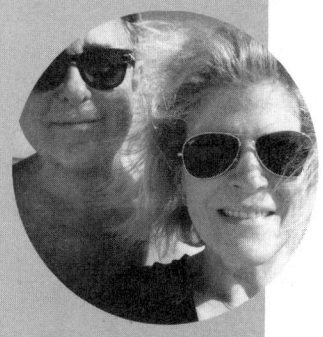

No more excuses. The perfect moment is, and will always be, right now.

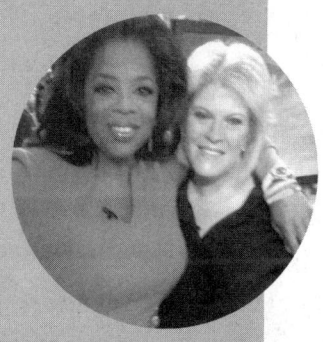

31

A Marathon, Not a Sprint

O n the weekend we get back from Miami, an interview in the *New York Times* with Karen May, Google's head of human resources, gives me new appreciation for the hurdle that Barbara faced when she talked to me and the unspoken dynamic between us at the time. May says that discussing any sensitive subject with an employee creates immediate tension and risks, "potentially leading them to feel worse about themselves ... it's difficult to tell somebody something that isn't working about them." Boy, can I relate.

That said, May favors telling people what they need to know, not what they want to hear. "If I'm not doing well ... and no one will tell me, I won't be able to fix it," she said. "And if you give me the information, the moment that the information is being transferred is painful, but then I have the opportunity to change it. I've come to realize that one of the most valuable things I could do for somebody is tell them exactly what nobody else has told them before." In my case, that was true: I needed to hear what everyone else was thinking. May said that 70 percent of employees do something to turn themselves around after being criticized, but the remainder can't because "they are either not willing to take it in, it doesn't fit their self-image, they're too resistant, in denial, or they don't have the wherewithal to change it." Obviously, I had been through numerous stages of denial, so I was ready to join the ranks of those who want to turn themselves around.

Finally—and most tellingly for me—May said that "change happens in small increments. So if you're watching to see if someone's changing, you have to watch for the incremental change. It's not a straight line." I appreciate Barbara even more after reading this because she clearly knows from her own experience that people change over time. She never expected me to shed fifty pounds by Easter. When I began to lose, she said something nice, and as I continued to drop in size, she kept the nice thoughts coming.

Two days later, it's New Year's Eve and we're staying home as usual, only this year I'm not even remotely thinking about celebrating with food as I did last year at this time, when all I could think about was my desperate need to eat a baked potato loaded with butter and perhaps some serious chocolate cake. I remember how miserable I was when I managed to control myself exactly one year ago. How far I've come. Peter makes some chicken cutlets along with vegetables and a salad—nothing out of the ordinary, in fact a fairly typical meal that we all enjoy.

Lying in bed waiting for the ball to drop in Times Square, I post on Facebook a photo of Emma and me wearing those goofy, glittery plastic glasses in the shape of 2013. My caption reads: "One of my proudest accomplishments of 2012: First full year ever without a single sip of soda. Only H_2O." Within an hour I get more than two hundred "likes" and dozens of congratulatory comments, plus plenty of posts asking how I've managed to stick to it.

Then I get this text from my Oklahoma pal Cindy, who just months ago told me she was desperate to lose weight but couldn't envision life without her daily glass or two of wine.

"OK, I'm ready," her text reads.

"Ready for what?" I ask, assuming she's referring to a big bash in Tulsa to ring in the New Year.

"I will give up the wine."

Sensing that she may indeed be ready, I push a bit further. "What about that diet Dr Pepper?"

"Yup, that too."

She's in—and I promise to be her best cheerleader.

"I want to experience what this so-called Shift is all about," her last text says. "Transform me, baby, I'm all yours."

A few minutes before the ball drops, my iPhone pings and it's an email from Nick, wishing me a happy New Year.

Fifteen years ago when I was a teenager, our fridge and cupboards were stocked with everything a growing boy wanted: Hot Pockets, Cheetos, cookies, and more. At some point you phased out those foods and I watched Atkins take over the house—steak 24/7 wasn't the worst thing. That was replaced (in no particular order) by diet capsules, sugar-free everything, grapefruits, and lots of other weird stuff that wasn't an appetizing snack after soccer practice. Everything always changed and nothing ever stuck. I always thought you were trying to fix a problem that was too complicated for any mainstream get-thin-quick solution.

But now, over the past year, I've seen you lose some weight, then more weight, and then a lot of weight. I don't know the specifics, but I imagine it took an amazing amount of willpower and an overall change in the way you view eating and living. The lesson I've learned from your incredible feat is that in order for deeply rooted change to happen, you can't rely on quick fixes. You have to stick to your guns. No cheating, no free passes. Stay strong until you reach your goal.

I've never seen you as anything but beautiful, but I'm so proud of you for reaching your longtime personal goal. Last time I was home, there were no diet gimmicks. All I found was a proud, confident, and healthy you—and that's all that matters to me. Here's to 2013! Love you, Nick.

It doesn't get much better: chops from a twenty-seven-year-old guy with a thirty-inch waist who thinks that he looks better in the Barbour jacket we gave him for Christmas than Daniel Craig does in *Skyfall*. Nick is a tough critic, but I've always valued his blunt honesty and the way he pulls no punches, no more so than now.

It doesn't matter whether you want to lose weight to save your career, to make yourself more attractive, to improve your health, or to break free from being burdened by your size. None of the reasons matter once you make the decision to make it happen. To make the Shift. What counts are the mini and massive rewards you get from taking charge of your life and finally acting on whatever is in you that you know must change. The process alone—just doing it—is an eye-opener, and you're bound to find a new appreciation for people and things you never noticed before. It's hard, yes, but you're absolutely worth it.

make the Shift

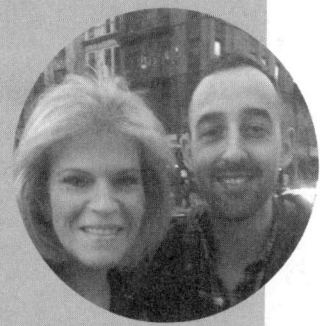

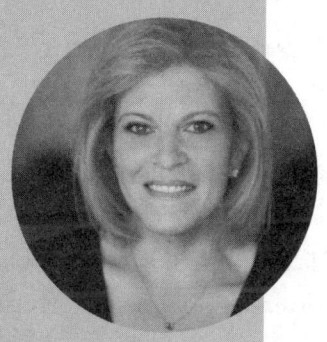

Don't rely solely on willpower, rely on inspiration. What is so important to you that you will do anything it takes to make this change?

Epilogue

t's New Year's morning and I'm ready for the big moment. This day starts like any other—peeing on a strip and standing on the scale—only today I'll learn what all my efforts in the past year have amounted to. I know I've lost a lot of weight, but now I'll find out exactly just how much. On January 1, 2012, I stashed a small note card in an envelope with a handwritten number on it. I open the top drawer of my dresser to pull it out. Only I know the number and it's seared in my mind, but I want to see it in print anyway. I tear open the envelope and the number is right there, in thick red Sharpie marker.

A three-digit number that once made me cringe.

How could I have ever let myself get so big? At times I

weighed more than Peter—and he's five inches taller than I am and a muscular man. But I remind myself that the number scribbled on the card is not a scarlet letter or, as I once thought, a prison sentence. The past is the past.

"Okay, I'm ready to do it," I say to him as he reads the *Times* in bed.

"Nervous?"

"So-so," I say.

The truth is my daily weigh-ins have given me a very good idea of what to expect, but I'm hoping for the absolute best. I slip off my sweats, pull the T-shirt over my head and drop it to the floor. I step on the scale. The needle shakes back and forth as it always does, then stops at the number in the center.

Another three-digit number. This one significantly smaller. One that if you had told me I could reach with a magical method called "the Shift," I would've followed you anywhere.

I quickly calculate how much I've lost in one year: sixty-two pounds. Whoa. That is a lot of weight, and my first thought is: *Great, you did it.* But almost immediately that switches to: *Gross, how could you have needed to lose that much?*

I stand on the scale for a few minutes, almost daring the needle to move. But it doesn't. I ask Peter to come into the bathroom, read the number, and see for himself.

"Sweetie, this is incredible," Peter says, kissing and hugging me while rubbing my back. "I am *so* happy for you."

"Hey, kids, get in here!" he calls loudly, as I get dressed. Sleepy-eyed Emma and Jake come into our bedroom, yawning, then they give me hugs too when they hear the news. For a few minutes I sit still on the edge of the bed marveling at my accomplishment—*sixty-two pounds*—until Peter calls me to the kitchen and says something that puts all the hard work of the past year in a new perspective.

"You know, it's interesting," he says. "Obviously sixty-two pounds is an enormous amount of weight for anyone to lose, no matter their size, and a terrific accomplishment. But if you look at how much you lost over the course of an entire year, it was just a little more than a pound a week."

"That's not very much," I say. "In fact, it's a lot less than I would have expected."

"Five point one six pounds a month," Jake calls from the living room couch.

Five pounds a month.

The number astounds me. I remember all my past attempts at slimming down and how I always rejected diets that did not promise *big* results in a short period of time. I wanted *instant* gratification, and I had no patience for any plan that promised a payoff over time. But now, as I continue to marvel at my number—*sixty-two*—I realize that two of the best-known clichés about weight loss are so true:

1. It *is* a marathon, not a sprint.
2. Slow and steady wins this race.

If I had known this before I started my journey—that all my work would result in my losing *only* five pounds a month—I probably would have given up. After all, I never set any weekly, monthly, or annual weight-loss goals. All I knew was that I was going to change my life and eating habits, and I was hell-bent on no longer being fat.

I mention it now because anyone making the Shift needs to know that small, consistent steps will lead to a big, cumulative payoff. You must be patient—and patience is something I never had before. You might not notice any difference week to week, but over the long haul if you stick to the pledge you have made to yourself, I promise you will. I am living proof of it.

If someone had told me one year ago that I could lose sixty-two pounds in one year simply by carefully watching what I ate, moving around more, standing on a scale each morning, and sticking with it, I would have gladly signed up.

But if you told me I could lose a pound or so a week, I'd probably have taken a pass. *A pound a week! This will take forever.*

As I look back on my journey, I realize that I made my Shift through five key steps. They all had much more to do with what was in my head than what I put in my mouth. It's a formula that you too can follow and make a significant change in your life as I did in mine.

STEP ONE: HOW FED UP ARE YOU, REALLY?

By this I mean: Are you finally sick of the status quo? I was. For the first time in my life, I recognized that the pain of being fat far outweighed the pain of changing. Yes, change is hard, but being fat is harder. When you're at a point when the pain of the present outweighs all the pain and sacrifice that change demands, you're ready to make the Shift.

STEP TWO: WHAT ARE YOU WILLING TO
GIVE UP?

Big change takes big sacrifice. No way around it. For me, that meant giving up a lot of things I once enjoyed a lot: sweet stuff, going to the movies, and frequent dinners out, just to name a few. Yet many people who want to lose weight or make other big changes resist committing to sacrifice and put up roadblocks that handicap any chance they have of succeeding before they even get started. They refuse to give up a nightly glass of wine, a cigarette after a stressful day, or a weekly pasta dinner. They promise to stick to a plan that they've outlined for themselves, then cheat at every turn. For the Shift to work for you, *nothing* can be more important than tackling your goal. You must give up things that once seemed near and dear to you, but have actually contributed to your struggles, such as poor foods and destructive behavior. You must accept the Shift as an all-or-nothing deal, as hard as it sounds. And it is hard, but it becomes easier to live with in time.

STEP THREE: WHAT'S YOUR PLAN?

There's no winging it when you're serious about making a significant shift in your life. You need to spell out clear, concise rules for yourself to eliminate ambiguity. Make a plan for how you're going to tackle your issue. For me, cutting carbs was the right method to lose weight because I knew from Day One what I could and couldn't eat. That made it simple for me, cut and dried, with no gray areas. I stuck with my plan and it paid off because I knew my parameters. Give yourself specific guidelines, put those steps in writing, and keep them close.

STEP FOUR: WHAT'S YOUR DAILY ACCOUNTABILITY?

It's easy to slip up when nobody's looking. It's also possible to fool yourself into thinking that you're on the straight and narrow when you're not. Daily weigh-ins are my reality check. For me, a watchful and loving family, changes in clothing size, feedback from colleagues, and photos are good secondary sources of accountability. Establish a system that works for you, so you can keep yourself honest and accountable, then stick to it.

STEP FIVE: HOW WILL YOU EMBRACE PATIENCE AND CELEBRATE YOUR VICTORIES?

Until I made the Shift, I was never patient or persistent enough to make a dent in my weight. I always gave up too soon for a variety of reasons, most of them bogus. I succeeded this time because *I viewed this Shift not as a diet but as a journey that was going to take time.* I forced myself to be both patient and persistent, not because I suddenly recognized that this was the way to go, but because I discovered early that overnight results were just not going to happen. I paused often—sometimes several times a day—before making hasty food choices that I knew I'd regret. To stay motivated, celebrate teeny victories often with proper rewards. An alcoholic should not celebrate a month of sobriety with a shot of whiskey, just as I don't think someone with a lifelong weight problem should reward herself for losing a few pounds with cake and chips. Figure out safe treats that will motivate you without derailing your long-term success.

Peter asked me today how hard it was. I thought about it for a few minutes before I told him it wasn't nearly as difficult as I thought it would be. Sure, it wasn't always fun or easy giving up bad habits and saying no to plenty of my favorite foods, but in retrospect it was all doable. Did I fall into a funk from time to time? Yes, but only when I failed to tell myself that I was strong and I could do this. I did, and aside from the proudest moments of my life—marrying Peter and giving a shot at life to our two wonderful children—nothing comes close to the sense of pride and wonder that I feel about what I have done. I am a new woman, mentally and physically. With each and every day, the ghosts that haunted me since childhood recede further in my mind. It's only been a few months since my weight loss became significant, but it has brought an inner strength that is now part of who I am. It's not an act this time.

I'm not done with my journey—I don't think I ever will be—and actually I'd like to lose some more weight. For my immediate future I think about two rewards—one tangible, one less so—that will mark my achievement. First, I'm going to have a small charm made in the form of the number *62* that will hang from my gold bracelet. I'll wear that number now and forever to remind myself that when I want something badly enough, anything is possible. Second, tomorrow morning I'm calling my doctor, whom I haven't seen in more than ten years, to make an appointment for a checkup. I'm going to get a full workup, the whole nine yards, including my first mammogram.

I'll never again neglect my health, just as I'll never again be fat. I've made the Shift—and I'm good with that.

Your Turn to Shift

The Shift isn't just the story about the year that changed my body and, in the process, changed my life. It's a movement of self-care that is guiding thousands of women toward their happiest, healthiest self. Let's start talking and let's help each other. Connect with me at **ShiftwithTory.com**, where you'll find advice, resources, recipes, and community, along with specific links to join me and our collective conversation for inspiration and encouragement on Facebook.com/Tory; Twitter.com/Tory Johnson; pinterest.com/Tory Johnson; and Instagram.com/Tory Johnson.

Remember: The perfect moment to start is, and will always be, *right now.*